PHARMACEUTICAL ETHICS and HEALTH CARE ACCESS

Richard George Boudreau

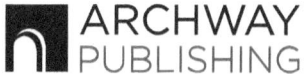

Archway Publishing books may be ordered through booksellers or by contacting:

Archway Publishing
1663 Liberty Drive
Bloomington, IN 47403
www.archwaypublishing.com
844-669-3957

ISBN: 978-1-6657-0568-4 (sc)
ISBN: 978-1-6657-0566-0 (hc)
ISBN: 978-1-6657-0567-7 (e)

Library of Congress Control Number: 2021907604

Print information available on the last page.

Archway Publishing rev. date: 05/05/2021

CONTENTS

ABSTRACT

Turing Pharmaceuticals/Vyera Pharmaceuticals' Martin Shkreli brought the problem of greedy US pharmaceutical companies into the public eye. This is because the company's move to increase the price of its drug Daraprim by enormous amounts was more the rule than the exception. Turing/Vyera is not alone in such outrageous price increases when it comes to pharmaceuticals sold in the United States. A fragmented industry, complete with manufacturers, pharmacy benefit managers, insurance companies, physicians, and pharmacists, combined with longer life expectancies is helping to push the price of drugs. These factors have been aided and abetted by a US government that lacks any kind of central authority for negotiating prices with pharmaceutical manufacturers, while providing the perfect environment for monopolistic practices and pricing. While pharmaceutical manufacturers point to increased costs of research and development for higher prices, the truth is Big Pharma, along with other industry stakeholders, operate in an environment of secrecy, with no rhyme or reason when it comes to charges.

The issue also brings up several ethical concerns, chief among them being how much should actually be charged for drugs (i.e., what is a "just" price) and whether the industry itself is behaving in an ethical fashion as it continues to increase costs. Though some cost increases are justified, the problem is that overpriced drugs are affecting vulnerable populations and US society as a whole. While the current and future presidents of the United States have provided plans and ideas to lower drug prices, not much can be done without specific, legislative enforcement, which is not likely to be coming any time soon.

It doesn't have to be that way, however. Other countries have been able to initiate price controls, overseen by central authorities, to help keep costs in check. It will, however, require a concerted effort among legislators, pharmaceutical industry stakeholders, doctors, pharmacists, and consumers. Only understanding that higher pharmaceutical prices come from myriad and complex factors can help us take better control of what is happening.

INTRODUCTION

In 2015, New York City entrepreneur Martin Shkreli made headlines, and not in a good way. As CEO of Turing Pharmaceuticals (now Vyera Pharmaceuticals), Shkreli had acquired Daraprim (the generic name is pyrimethamine), an antiparasite medication useful for treating toxoplasmosis, especially among patients with HIV (Hamblin 2015). This wasn't the problem. Many pharmaceutical manufacturers, as we'll see in this paper, buy drugs from other companies or actually buy companies that manufacture drugs.

What put Shkreli in the eye of the media and drove him into the court of negative public opinion was that he increased the price of this drug from $13.50 to $750 (Hamblin 2015). Adding insult to injury, Shkreli showed no remorse or shame when it came to the price increase (nor did he really indicate a reason for it). Rather, his sneering, arrogant response to public outrage earned him the nickname "Pharma Bro," positioning him as a poster boy of apparent pharmaceutical industry greed (Owles 2017). While Shkreli wasn't, at the time, the only pharmaceutical executive to raise prices for no apparent reason on a drug, he was the most visible. This in turn made him an ideal target by the media and general public for blame of overall high prices from pharmaceuticals.

Adding to the problem, he didn't help himself with his response. Rather than facing his critics with calm, reasoned logic for the price increase, Shkreli taunted his critics via television interviews and Twitter as well as taking his self-serving rant to YouTube, where he posted hour-long, livestream, rambling commentary, which only served to promote even angrier backlash.

Shkreli was eventually brought up on charges—not for jacking up the price of Daraprim but for eventual securities fraud. Ironically enough, three years after the incident, Vyera Pharmaceuticals continued to price Daraprim at more than $750 per pill (Luthra 2018). This, even as the notorious Pharma Bro began serving his seven-year sentence for securities fraud (Long and Hays 2018). In other words, despite public shaming, not much had changed. Nor, it's likely, will it.

Shefali Luthra with KHN noted in 2018,

> The continued high price of the drug is a cautionary tale to those who hope that public shaming of a few "bad actors" can curb escalating drug prices, because the problem is rooted in the market's underlying financial incentives.

In other words, Shkreli and Vyera aren't the only "bad actors" when it comes to high pharmaceutical prices. The entire industry is filled with people like Shkreli. The difference is these individuals are better at keeping quiet or responding more logically whenever they increase prices on drugs for no apparent reason.

The story with Vyera isn't over, however. Part of the issue involved with the 2015 price increase was that even while Daraprim's patent expired, both for the drug and its active ingredient—it had already been on the market for several decades—no generic equivalent, surprisingly, had been introduced, at least not in the United States (Luthra 2018).

This opened another can of worms. In late January 2020, the Federal Trade Commission filed charges against Vyera Pharmaceuticals, claiming that the company struck deals with distributors to prevent generic companies from obtaining samples and sales data for Daraprim (Dearment 2020b). Even to anyone who doesn't know much about how the pharmaceutical industry operates, this type of action is definitely against any kind of antitrust law. The result was that a month later, the Food and Drug Administration (FDA) announced it had approved the first generic version of Daraprim (pyrimethamine), which would be manufactured by New York-based Cerovene (FDA 2020b). As of now, however, it's not certain how much the generic drug will cost, and Cerovene is remaining tight-lipped about the price.

It is true that Daraprim (and its potential generic equivalent) is used to treat a relatively small percentage of the US population. A large part of the population, fortunately, doesn't suffer from toxoplasmosis. The Daraprim story, however, is a very good example of the mess known as the US pharmaceutical industry. Within this industry, out-of-control prices are set amid secrecy and within a monopolistic environment operating under the tacit approval of the federal government. To repeat, the industry has any number of Shkrelis who increase prices on drugs simply because they can.

Or because they want to please shareholders. Or for any number of reasons that have little to do with the actual cost of researching, manufacturing, and distributing a drug.

The unfortunate issue, however, is that these higher prices end up hurting a variety of demographics who struggle to afford the medicine they need.

High prescription drugs are a main reason as to why patients don't take their prescribed medications (Fiscella et al. 2019). This in turn results in avoidable emergency department visits and hospitalizations. Additionally, high prescription costs put patients in a difficult predicament as they have to decide between paying for rent, food, and other bills and paying for their much-needed drugs.

Another unfortunate issue is that, while it's easy to point the finger at the Pharma Bro, his company, and his colleagues, it isn't just the pharmaceutical industry that is the problem. Big Pharma—a collection of the larger pharmaceutical manufacturers—is only part of the reason for out-of-control costs. This is one reason why, in the past, simply passing legislation or attempting to "shame" the pharmaceutical companies (which is, in fact, what President Donald Trump tried to do) doesn't have much impact on the problem.

According to Axene Health Partners,

> The current pharmaceutical market structure is a combination of patent-protected brand-name drugs, where manufacturing is controlled by the firm holding the patent, and generic drugs, where the exclusive patent has expired, and any manufacturer meeting minimum requirements may produce the drug.

As such, the difficulty currently being faced is that, for the most part, ad hoc or knee-jerk decisions are being made, which don't really end up solving the main problems involving prescription drug prices (van der Gronde, Uyl-de Groot, and Pieters 2017).

This, in part, is the problem when it comes to high pharmaceutical costs and solutions in lowering them. The amount that patients pay for a brand-name drug depends on a variety of factors, ranging from the insurance plan to the plan's formulary, the size of the deductible, and the deal the insurance company has worked out with the pharmaceutical manufacturer (Entis 2019). Regardless of which entity in the vast supply chain is at fault for the high prices, the system isn't designed to prioritize savings for patients.

This means finding a solution can't be a one-size-fits-all focus. Rather, the solutions require an understanding of the complex issues that drive this trend. Once understood, solutions can be proposed to help reign in prices and to help ensure that prescription meds are created—and distributed—in a more balanced and ethical manner.

In this book, I'll propose some solutions to consider. First, however, I'll outline how we got into the current mess we're in today, where exactly we are, and why. I'll focus on the industry players and their roles in what is being charged. I'll also examine the ethics of the situation, given that the pharmaceutical industry is an important part of the overall health care industry—also a mess in the United States, by the way—a discussion about ethics, and value to society is warranted.

With the clear issue and factors in front, I'll propose some thoughts and solutions to the scenario.

Solving the problem of high pharmaceutical costs won't be easy.

But if all stakeholders involved can get together and do their part, it can be done. The question, of course, is whether the solutions proposed can be enacted. My belief is that, as it stands, anything involving legislation or federal control is not going to be completed any time soon. Because of this, it's up to the end user—both health care providers who write prescriptions for the drugs as well as the patients who take those drugs—to take their own steps to ensure that drug prices remain affordable.

HISTORY: BUILDING BLOCKS OF HIGH PRICES

AS WITH EVERYTHING TO DO WITH HIGH COSTS IN ANY
part of US health care, high costs of pharmaceuticals didn't happen
overnight. Nor has there been only one reason for where we are now.
Unsurprisingly, there are several factors behind the current causes.
According to Anthony A. Barrueta, Kaiser Permanente's senior vice
president of government relations (2015), the more recent timeline
concerning out-of-control pricing in the pharmaceutical industry is
as follows:

- 1988: The Medicare Catastrophic Coverage Act (MCCA)
  improves acute care benefits for the elderly.
- 1990: The Omnibus Budget Reconciliation Act (OBRA 90)
  establishes Medicaid best price, killing off discounting and
  even negotiating.
- 1995: The Uruguay Round Agreements Act extends patent
  protection from seventeen years to twenty years from date
  of first filing of patent application, allowing pharmaceutical
  companies more monopolies.

- 1997: The FDA strengthens direct-to-consumer (DTC) advertising from drug companies; this leads to an increase of television and magazine ads promoting pharmaceuticals.
- 2003: The Medicare Modernization Act (MMA) adds Part D to Medicare while also stressing noninterference of Medicare when it comes to negotiating drug prices.
- 2007: The oral chemotherapy parity law trend begins. States begin passing legislation mandating the coverage of oral chemotherapy (by June 2014, thirty-four states and DC have laws on the books); while providing more efficiency in at-home chemotherapy treatments, this also effectively increases the price of such treatment.
- 2010: The Affordable Care Act (ACA) institutes out-of-pocket limits on spending for consumers, though pharmaceuticals aren't included on many plans, especially Medicare.
- 2014: Gilead introduces Sovaldi/Harvoni, a highly expensive drug formulated and released to treat hepatitis C; I will discuss Solvadi's $84,000 price tag later on in this paper.

Barrueta was absolutely correct with his timeline in that the US experienced higher pharmaceutical costs, due to factors launched in the late 1980s. However, while the late 1980s and 1990s are considered the time during which pharmaceutical prices really began taking off, it's also important to understand the history of pharmaceuticals, how they shaped the US health care system, and how—and why—they ended up becoming as expensive as they are now.

◆ In the Beginning

The origin of the word *drug,* is likely Arabic, though no one actually knows. What we do know is that the first reference to *drug* appeared in Old German as *drog,* which referred to a type of powder (Jones 2011). We know a little more about the etymology of the word *toxicology,* which comes from the Greek word *toxikos,* literally referring to a bow used for shooting arrows. At the time, and even sooner, early hunters learned the art of spiking darts and arrows with poisons from plants to kill or temporarily maim wild prey—hence, toxikos.

These days, of course, toxicology is the study of the impact of chemicals on living organisms. Those "chemicals," in many cases, can be considered the pharmaceuticals fighting living organisms, from cancer cells to dangerous bacteria. Chemotherapy in a sense is poison; it destroys cancer cells as well as live cells.

Going back to the very early days of *drogs,* many of the first pharmaceuticals were natural in that they came from plants, herbs, and shrubs as well as insects and reptiles. Pharmacologically active substances coming from plants include opium (from poppies), nicotine (from tobacco plants), cannabinoids (from cannabis leaves), cardiac glycosides (from foxglove), and quinine (from the cinchona tree) (Jones 2011; Weatherall 1990). It was not unusual for cave dwellers, and then early agrarian societies, to experiment with different plants and insects in an effort to prevent or mitigate disease (Jones 2011). However, many of those early societies also attributed disease and illness to spiritual reasons as opposed to changes in body chemistry. It wasn't really until the age of reason, during which doctors were considered more than individuals who drove out evil spirits, that it was realized that some diseases could be treated without resorting to prayer. As such, the medicinal use of plants and herbs continued throughout the seventeenth century, though isolating and characterizing the active principles in these plants proved to be a major challenge for chemists at the time (Jones 2011). Actually, it wasn't until the scientific revolution of the seventeenth century—and its spread of rationalism and experimentation—that the industry as we know it today took off (PharmaPhorum 2020).

◆ From Apothecaries to Research and Development

While in the early days people would gather their own leaves and insects with which to make medicines, alchemists (who later become apothecaries) could be considered the forerunners of both modern pharmaceutical manufacturers and pharmacists. These alchemists/apothecaries, with their skills in herbology and toxicology, knew how to gather ingredients and then make all types of herbal remedies in hopes of finding a cure for medical complaints (Jones 2011). It probably goes without saying that treating a patient involved a great deal of trial and error.

Fredrich Sertuner (1783–1841) was considered the first to succeed in separating beneficial healing chemicals from a plant, as he isolated a plant alkaloid into a pure state. This eventually came to be known as morphine. He was able to do this by isolating meconic acid from raw opium; when the base of this was administered to a dog, the animal fell into a deep sleep. Not long afterward, other alkaloids were separated and isolated from opium; one of these was codeine.

By the mid-1800s, German scientists began dominating the field of analytical and organic chemistry. The major focus of these chemists and early toxicologists was to develop methods allowing the identification of plant alkaloids in blood and human viscera, more to determine poisoning as opposed to healing or treating diseases. The first synthetic drugs—again, the field of German organic chemists—were discovered and modified in the 1800s, with Justus von Liebig discovering chloroform, which eventually was important in its use as a general anesthetic drug by Scottish physician James Young Simpson.

The growth in this form of chemistry led to the field of pharmacology. This was established as a scientific discipline by the latter part of the nineteenth century. One of the first German chemical firms demonstrating an interest in these pharmaceuticals and ending up producing many of the earlier known synthetic drugs was the Friedrich Bayer Company, founded in 1863. Interestingly enough, the company's early success was focused on seeking out chemicals in waste products from dye works, leading to mild analgesics (and eventually aspirin) (Jones 2011). In fact, many roots of the early pharmaceutical industry can be traced to chemicals that were, at one point, used for dyes.

By the eighteenth and early nineteenth centuries, both chemical research and pharmacology advanced to the point during which drugs included the following (McCarthy 2017):

- anodynes (pain relievers): opium and laudanum (opium, saffron, and Canary wine)
- anti-arthritics: Epsom salts and cinchona

- antidysenterics: ipecac and paregoric
- antipyrectics (for fever): emetics, cinchona, laxatives, and cold baths
- emetics (to induce vomiting to treat food poisoning): tartar emetic, ipecac, and honey
- muscle relaxers: opium, wine, cinchona, and oil of amber
- intestinal irritation purgatives or cathartics: Glauber's salt, plumbers' pills, ipecac, jalap, calomel, salme, rhubarb, castor oil, and Epsom salts
- sudorifics or diaphoretics (to induce perspiration): camphor, Dover's powder (opium and ipecac), and rhubarb
- diuretics (to treat edema by increasing urine flow): milk, dandelion extract, juniper berries, and lemon juice

The advent of the Industrial Revolution led to the mass production of goods; pharmaceuticals and drugs were no different. In 1827, Henrich Emanuel Merck began manufacturing and selling alkaloids in bulk (PharmaPhorum 2020). Beecham (now GlaxoSmithKline) began producing patented medicines in 1842 and built the world's first factory for producing only pharmaceuticals in 1859. Pfizer, founded in 1849 by German immigrants as a fine-chemicals business, found their business expanding rapidly during the Civil War as demand for painkillers and antiseptics increased. Eli Lilly, a colonel serving in the Union Army during the Civil War, eventually set up a pharmaceutical business in 1876, being one of the first to focus on R&D as well as manufacturing.

Then came a way for these chemicals to be distributed to the general public. The roots of American pharmacies came from English shops, wholesalers, and general stores (McCarthy 2017). While almost all medicines were imported from England, the Revolutionary War led to the development of domestic sources of medicine. During the seventeenth century, these drugs could be found in general stores as part of multipurpose dispensaries.

At the time, apothecarists were, in a sense, physicians. They would diagnose issues and diseases and then prepare medical products. The pharmacists or druggists owned the dispensaries, and most of these pharmacists relied on materia medica, a collection of the therapeutic properties of medicine later to be known as pharmacology. Prescriptions were not needed in those days simply because the medical profession was vastly different from the one we confront today.

Jonathan Roberts, America's first hospital "pharmacist," was actually an apprentice physician, as were most of the early hospital pharmacists. Roberts's successor suggested separating the pharmacy and medical practices; by 1822, the New York Hospital employed a full-time pharmaceutical practitioner. While most people were treated at home during the nineteenth century, the demand for hospital pharmacists increased during the War between the States. Pharmacists were individuals with expertise in drug preparation manufacturing and in buying drugs. During the early 1800s, physicians began writing prescriptions for apothecaries to compound and dispense. Between 1820 and 1860, the practice of pharmacy was officially split off from the practice of medicine, with the two practices requiring different skills and education.

An increase in immigration to the US in the late 1800s also led to an increased demand for hospitals and hospital pharmacists.

Hospitals realized it was more cost-effective to fill prescriptions in-house rather than by using community pharmacies. While standards and pharmaceutical requirements were proposed during the late nineteenth century, it wasn't until the early twentieth century that specific legislation and laws were passed to protect the general public from "quack" medicine. These included the Biologics Control Act of 1902 and the original Pure Food and Drugs Act of 1906 (FDA). World War I meant advancement of health care and surgical techniques on the field. It wasn't until after the first World War, however, that the pharmaceutical industry really took shape, becoming the forerunner of what we are used to today.

◆ The World Wars and Their Aftermath

Between World War I and World War II, one major competitive strategy among the pharmaceutical companies was research. Before the wars, the focus of these companies (many of which started life as chemical manufacturers) was development and distribution. However, many of the pharmaceutical companies, during the inter-war years, established in-house laboratories while forging collaborative relationships with academic, biomedical, chemical, and clinical researchers through grants-in-aid and fellowships (Tobbell, 2012).

For example, in 1935, I. G. Farbenindustrie of Germany discovered sulfanilamide, an anti-infective agent, while screening dyes for antimicrobial activity. Following this discovery, industrial and academic researchers began screening both chemical and natural compounds for antimicrobial activity, leading to the isolation of hundreds of different antibiotic agents (including penicillin) in 1940.

The development of these drugs launched what was considered a "therapeutic revolution." For the first time, physicians had drugs that could cure patients of infections, rather than simply relieving symptoms. Penicillin was discovered by Alexander Fleming in the late 1920s. However, a government-supported international collaboration made up of Merck, Pfizer and Squibb set up functions to mass produced the drug during World War II (PharmaPhorum, 2020).

Also developed during this period was insulin, for treatment of diabetes. In finding this particular drug, chemist Frederick Banting was able to isolate materials to treat insulin deficiency, leading to problems with high blood sugar. But it was only in collaboration with scientists at Eli Lilly that he and his colleagues both purified the extract and produced and distributed it as an effective medicine.

However, despite early regulations, the trade in medicines and drugs was highly unregulated, meaning a less strict delineation between "pharmaceutical" and "chemical" industries. One good example of this was Bayer's loss of its Aspirin trademark; the company had its assets seized during World War I, while Merck was split off from its German parent company. That loss of trademark is why these days "aspirin" is a generic designation rather than a branded one.

One major transformation of the US pharmaceutical industry took place between the 1930s and 1950s, during which the industry went from one dominated by small and medium companies specializing in the bulk manufacture of fine chemicals, or the wholesale production of pharmaceuticals, to an industry dominated by several fully integrated companies, complete with extensive research facilities, growing medical departments and marketing capabilities. These changes came about due to changes in more sophisticated research and regulatory environments. As mentioned above, federal statutes only loosely regulated pharmaceuticals on the market (Gregory, 2016). This changed in 1938 when Congress enacted the Federal Food, Drug and Cosmetics Act, requiring manufacturers to submit data regarding the safety of a new drug before it entered the consumer marketplace.

Furthermore, during World War II, the Committee on Medical Research of the Office of Scientific Research and Development contracted with drug companies to develop penicillin, antimalarial drugs, steroids, and replacement blood products and the companies themselves used existing connections with academic researchers to meet wartime demands. This confirmed the value of corporate research, and following the end of World War II, the pharmaceutical companies increased research facilities and staff.

These new antibiotic agents led to many drugs with similar therapeutic effects being introduced to the market. Because these drugs essentially did the same thing, the companies built intensive marketing efforts to build market share for the drugs.

Following the end of World War II, the pharmaceutical industry consisted of two types of core companies. There were the producers of fine chemicals, which bulk-manufactured chemical intermediates and active pharmaceutical agents in drug productions (these were known as the "fine chemicals") and then sold them to the second type of core company, the pharmaceutical companies. Merck and Pfizer were the largest of the fine chemical manufacturers, while Abbott Laboratories, Parke-Davis & Co., Smith, Kline & French, Squibb, Upjohn, and Eli Lilly made up what was then known as the "old-line pharmaceutical companies." The pharmaceutical companies would acquire active compounds from the chemical manufacturers, package them as drugs, and then sell them under their own trade/brand names to physicians, pharmacists, and hospitals. Because the Abbots, Quibbs, and Eli Lillys were, in a sense, responsible for marketing the drugs, they maintained small staffs who had the responsibility of selling the drugs to pharmacists, physicians, and hospitals (Tobbell, 2012). The fine chemical manufacturers, however, lacked any kind of significant marketing organization.

Also at this time, a shift in product production took place. More of the old-line pharmaceutical firms began to produce their own fine chemicals in-house, directly competing against Pfizer and Merck. Meanwhile, the fine chemical manufacturers were themselves producing their own innovative pharmaceutical compounds, but because they lacked the marketing capacity to market the drugs themselves, they still sold the active ingredients to the pharmaceutical companies that, in turn, packaged and marketed them under their own names. As such, during the 1950s, Pfizer built up its marketing organization while Merck merged with pharmaceutical company Sharp & Dohme.

◆ Price Fixing and Other Problems

Due to more resources committed to research and development, more drugs were introduced, such as those to control hypertension. As such, the 1940s and 1950s were considered decades of intense innovation by the American drug industry. This was also the period of time during which the United States replaced the German pharmaceutical industry as the leading pharmaceutical innovator in the world.

Adding to this was assistance from generous government funding. For instance, the National Institutes of Health saw its federal funding increase to nearly $100 million by 1956, an investment that helped fuel development of new drugs among the growing industry (PharmaPhorum, 2020).

However, as the industry became wealthier, perhaps unsurprisingly, concerns began to arise about potential ethical conflicts of making money from selling health care products. George Merck addressed the issue in 1950, pointing out, "We try never to forget that medicine is for the people. It is not for the profits."

Realizing that it was operating within the highly visible arena of health care, the pharmaceutical industry's leadership realized that it would need to build not just scientific networks but also relationships with health care practitioners (such as physicians) and pharmacists as well as the American public. The industry, at the time, promote itself as "a critical national asset in the global war against communism." This indirectly led to potential criticisms of government price controls. The argument was that any challenge to a system of free enterprise would lead to socialism, especially if the government interfered.

However, all was not wonderful amid these companies and their wonder drugs. By the mid-1950s, Merck, Pfizer, and other pharmaceutical companies were accused of fixing the prices of antibiotics and vaccines as well as engaging in misleading marketing practices. In 1959, Senator Estes Kefauver launched his Senate Subcommittee on Antitrust and Monopoly investigation into alleged administered pricing in the drug industry. Kefauver's concern was that drug prices weren't being determined by the market and fluctuations in supply and demand but were under control by the companies that held the patents—a monopoly—on the specific drugs. The Kefauver hearings launched what would become two decades' worth of congressional investigations into the business and pricing practices of the US drug industry.

By the time Kefauver began his investigation into the pharmaceutical industry, the so-called "free market" approach to medical innovation definitely had its costs (Greene and Podolsky, 2012). Insulin had been developed in the 1920s. Following seventeen months during which pharmaceutical executives were shown as profiteering and doctors were "portrayed as dupes of pharmaceutical companies' marketing departments," Kefauver presented his bill. The better-known components of the legislation focused on ensuring review claims by the US Food and Drug Administration (FDA) of efficacy prior to drug approval, along with monitoring of pharmaceutical advertising and ensuring that all drugs had readable generic names.

Kefauver's bill also proposed a compulsory licensing provision so that all important new drugs would generate competitive markets after three years. The senator also wanted to eliminate the so-called "me-too drugs," along with "molecular modifications," by insisting that a new drug be granted a patent only if it produced a therapeutic effect that was much greater than that of the drug before it was modified.

However, by the time the bill made its way through the subcommittee (and the trade associations), the bill was watered down. Kefauver continued insisting that compulsory licensing and patents be retained in the legislation, but his stubbornness cost him the bill.

In June 1962, officials from the Kennedy administration, backed by the pharmaceutical industry, presented the subcommittee with an alternate bill, which had no patent regulatory language. Kefauver claimed foul, the Kennedy administration dropped its support of S. 1552, and it was considered dead until the thalidomide scandal and its following outcry, which forced both Kefauver and Kennedy to support the gutted bill. This paper will focus on the thalidomide scandal in more detail later on; suffice it to say that the problems it caused shaped legislation concerning the safety and testing of new drugs.

The amendments granted the FDA power to demand proof of efficacy before approving new drugs for the US market as well as putting into play a retrospective review of drugs approved between 1938 and 1962. By the early 1970s, the Drug Efficacy Study Implementation program had categorized approximately six hundred medicines as "ineffective" and forced their removal from the market. However, one unintended consequence of the amendments was that pharmaceutical research needed to be organized around placebo-controlled and randomized controlled trials to help researchers gauge the efficacy of an individual drug. However, it made collecting such data much more difficult and much more expensive.

◆ Getting over Ulcers

By 1960, twenty pharmaceutical firms accounted for 80 percent of all US sales (Tobbell, 2012). However, the majority of pharmaceutical firms, other than the major ones, such as Merck and Lilly, did little research or promotion, but focused on packaging and distribution of unpatented or off-patent generic drugs; these firms were typically referred to as generic drug manufacturers. While research-based drug firms operated nationally and internationally, generic manufacturers were geographically dispersed, often operating on a state or regional level.

The drugs produced by these companies paid well but didn't have huge profit margins. This all changed when it came to answering the question as to how to treat peptic ulcers.

Peptic ulcers these days are considered more of a nuisance than the life-threatening disease it was. This is, in part, thanks to medications on the market as well as nutritional and other lifestyle changes.

Things were very different in the mid-twentieth century, however. Peptic ulcers were created by release of excess stomach acid, resulting in tears in the lining of the intestines. The most common treatment involved antacids, rest, and bland diets; in extreme cases, surgery could be performed. But left untreated, such ulcers could lead to severe bleeding or even death. At the very least, this disease was unpleasant and definitely had an impact on quality of life. Patients—and the market—were ready for something that could take care of it.

During the mid-1960s, a research team at Smith Kline & French Laboratories in the United Kingdom began research on a project to determine the physiology of acid secretion and to find a substance capable of blocking such effects (Molinder, 1994). The team believed that histamine was the final mediator of acid secretion and eight years later published evidence of burimamide, the first histamine2-receptor antagonist (unlike histimaine1 more commonly found in allergies) in treatment of excess release of acid. Additional research led to the creation of cimetidine, which was proven to effectively block acid secretions ultimately leading to and exacerbating ulcers. The product was ultimately marketed under the brand name of Tagamet. Tagamet was approved in the UK in 1976 for treatment of peptic ulcers and was released in the US in 1977 (PharmaPhorum, 2020).

The drug became enormously popular. More than a million patients in the United Kingdom, for example, were prescribed Tagamet during its first five years on the market (Pratt, 2017). During its seventeen years under patent protection, the drug generated $14 billion for Smith Kline & French (now part of GlaxoSmithKline). In addition to introducing a new way in which drugs were manufactured, Tagamet proved to be the first blockbuster drug—classified as such because its revenues topped $1 billion.

The high revenues and large profit marketing didn't last. Competition in the form of Zantac was eventually approved, and when Tagamet went off patent in 1994, both it and Zantac experienced declines in revenues. However, the search was on as drug manufacturers suddenly competed to become the developers of the next large blockbuster drugs. This ultimately led to the production of Prozac in 1987 by Eli Lilly and the first statin manufactured by Merck (PharmaPhorum, 2020). Also in this category are AbbVie's anti-inflammatory medication, Humira, and the hepatitis C drug Solvadi manufactured by Gilead. As we'll see later on in this paper, Solvadi has ended up the most expensive drug on the market, coming in at $84,000 for twelve weeks of treatment.

◆ The '90s and Price Increases

According to a study published in *Health Affairs,* US spending on pharmaceuticals took off in the late 1990s, tripling between 1997 and 2007 (Aitken, Berndt, and Cutler, 2008). The 1990s are generally recognized as the turning point for hugely escalating drug prices in the United States, mainly because a record number of new drugs were released during that decade (Frakt, 2018). Specifically, high-cost blood pressure medications and cancer drugs were released, a result of "the scientific explosion of the 1970s and 1980s, that allowed us to isolate the genetic basis of certain diseases," which in turn helped open "a lot of therapeutic new areas for new drugs," Harvard Medical School Associate Professor Aaron Kesselheim told the *New York Times.*

Also during that period, regulations on television drug advertising were relaxed, meaning more advertising, combined with an increase in FDA approvals, fueled by new fees collected from pharmaceutical manufacturers. This in turn added to the sudden increase of drugs coming to the market, as well as the overwhelmingly higher prices of drugs. Various studies have been conducted, focusing on pharmaceutical advertising and an increase in drug pricing. One study, focused on brands in five therapeutic classes, noted that advertising increased demand for those drugs, thereby also increasing sales for those therapeutic classes. In addition to increasing demand, increases in operating costs due to higher promotional spending is generally shifted to consumers, leading to higher prices (Dave, 2010).

Drug price increases did slow down in the 2000s, mainly attributed to a boost in generics drugs, along with fewer FDA approvals of blockbuster drugs. Then in 2014, drug prices began spiking again, possibly due to expensive specialty drugs for diseases such as hepatitis C and cystic fibrosis. Additionally, many of the new drugs are based on recent advances in science, such as completion of the human genome project. Because these are biologics, there is little competition, which means that these newer drugs command relatively higher prices. Biologics differ from pharmaceuticals in that the former is derived from biological methods (which might include living cells, requiring additional testing and clinical trials). Pharmaceuticals, on the other hand, are chemically based.

Biologic or pharmaceuticals, the fact that drugs were overpriced all came to a head with the advent of Daraprim and Martin Shkreli. The question, however, was whether the spotlight has done anything to really affect drug prices.

WHERE WE ARE NOW

THESE DAYS, THE US COULD BE CONSIDERED THE PHAR-
maceutical capital of the world (Prihoda, 2017). Four out of the
top ten growing pharmaceutical companies are headquartered in
the US, while the US develops more drugs than any other nation
(Prihoda, 2017; Jurney, 2016). Research and studies also prove that
Americans consume more drugs than almost any other developed
nation.

In addition to demonstrating a higher drug consumption,
Americans spend a lot more money on their drugs. According to a
report released by the US House Committee on Ways and Means,
Americans on average pay nearly four times more for drugs than
other countries; in some cases, they can pay sixty-seven times more
than other countries for the same drug (House Committee on Ways
and Means, 2019). At last count, according to the Organization for
Economic Co-operation and Development (OCED), Americans
spend $1,228.66 annually, per capita, on pharmaceuticals (OCED,
2019).

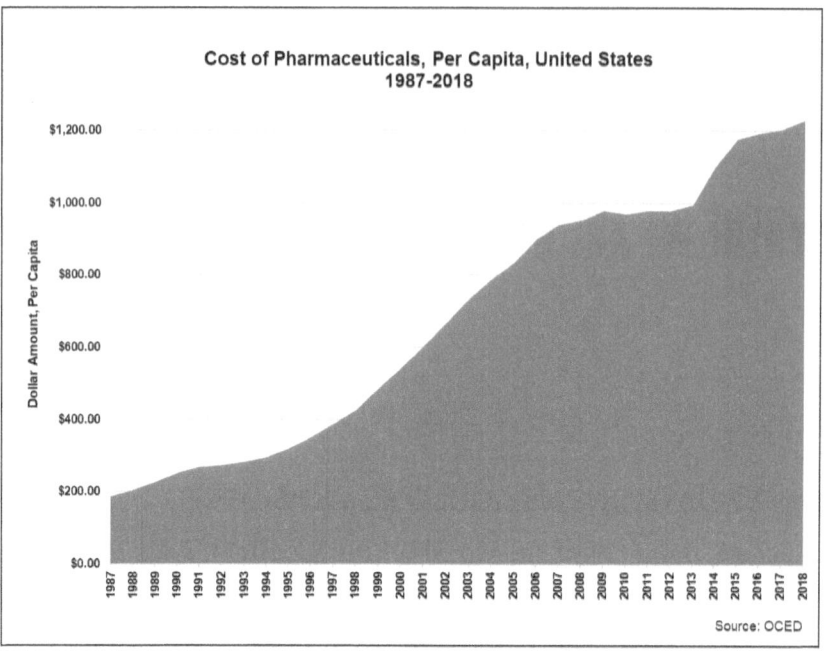

A 2018 report issued by the Department of Health and Human Services Office of the Inspector General underlined this assertion, reporting that the net spending on brand-name drugs in Medicare Part D increased 62 percent from 2011 to 2015 (Sarpatwari, DeBello, Zakarian, Najafzadeh, and Kesselheim, 2019). This occurred despite a 17 percent decrease in the number of prescriptions of these products over the same period of time.

And the costs of those drugs keep increasing (despite the Pharma Bro scandal and others we'll explore later on). A *Consumer Reports* survey, conducted in September 2019, indicated that 30 percent of Americans who currently take prescription medications indicated that out-of-pocket costs for a drug they regularly use increased from the year before (Gill, 2020). Of that representative survey involving

1,015 US adults, 12 percent reported that their drug costs increased by $100 or more (Gill, 2020).

Taking this another step, those who experienced spikes in out-of-pocket costs were almost twice as likely not to fill a prescription, forgo additional medical treatments or tests, cut back on groceries, or to get a second job. Not filling a prescription or cutting back on taking a particular drug to save money can cause consequences leading to further negative impacts on the US health care system.

Approximately two-thirds of the US pharmaceutical spending comes from private insurance, as well as out-of-pocket spending (Prihoda, 2017). The US government is paying approximately the same amount, per capita, as other OECD nations. Meanwhile, American consumers are being asked to pay, yet again, through private insurance premiums and out-of-pocket costs, meaning they are effectively being double charged when it comes to taking pills and medication.

If this wasn't enough, new drugs—which are sometimes questionable—continue being added to the market. It is the continued launch of so-called "novel" pharmaceuticals with high launch prices/price tags that add to overpricing of drugs. In 2017, the median annual list price of a new cancer medication was $160,000, compared to $101,000 in 2013 (Sarpatwari, DeBello, Zakarian, Najafzadeh, and Kesselheim, 2019). There are also routine price increases for existing products, accounting for about 60 percent of the boost in US revenues for forty-five top-selling drugs between 2014 and 2017. Adding even more injury to the above insult, there is no federal law or regulation keeping drug prices in check (Gill, 2020).

The questions then are these: Why can't we simply wave a magic wand and bring prices down? Or why Congress can't pass laws to keep better tabs on drug prices and approvals?

One reason is because efforts to reform prescription drug prices and the market are often tangled with larger policy debates about overall health care financing and delivery (Augustine, Madhavan, and Nass, 2018). Other reasons focus on the fear that any government action involving price controls would stifle free-market movement as well as innovation and new discoveries. It is these arguments, in fact, that continue to stymie any kind of meaningful reforms. And leading it all are organizations whose sole purpose and reason for being is to protect pharmaceutical manufacturers and others in the industry. The large, research-based firms making up the core of the industry's trade associations include the American Drug Manufacturers Association (ADMA) and the American Pharmaceutical Manufacturers Association (APMA), and later on, the Pharmaceutical Manufacturers Association (PMA) (Tobbell, 2012). These organizations ensure that Big Pharma, and other stakeholders involved with the manufacture and distribution of drugs, continues to receive its very large slice of the overall health care pie. Anytime changes are suggested, these organizations do a good job of waging information campaigns explaining why the status quo should be maintained.

Another reason is that health care overall is financed by many players, such as the federal and state governments, private employers, unions, and even households.

Furthermore, the industry's manufacturing and distribution arms are highly diversified and complex, making any kind of meaningful price reform even more difficult. To gain a better understanding of the complexity regarding high spending on drugs and pharmaceuticals, it's a good idea to examine the chain of events involved with getting a drug from manufacturer to market. The order is as follows (Drettwan and Kjos, 2019):

- Pharmaceutical manufacturers research and develop drugs.
- The drugs are delivered to pharmacies by wholesale distributors.
- The drugs are obtained by patients from these pharmacies; costs can vary, based on drug plan coverage and the pharmacies themselves.

The above doesn't even get into the whole issue of pharmacy benefit managers, health care providers, drug negotiations, and other aspects involved with getting a product from a pharma manufacturer to the end consumer.

Today's pharmaceutical industry "has evolved into a supremely complex amalgam of regulators, developers and manufacturers, retailers, insurers, wholesalers, physicians, employers offering benefits, and intermediaries, including organizations referred to as pharmacy benefit managers" (Augustine, Madhavan, and Nass, 2018). Adding to the scenario is that many transactions between these entities are secret and opaque, making it difficult to follow the money and understand how much is being spent and where.

Because of this, and because of the stakeholders involved with the process of getting a drug from the originator to the end user, blaming one thing for high prices is somewhat absurd. In actuality, the following are all contributors to higher drug prices.

◆ Pharmaceutical Manufacturers

I'm listing this first because, in most cases, the first finger of blame for higher drug prices is pointed to Big Pharma, the nickname given to the world's pharmaceutical industry. Big Pharma is often considered the cause of the price-gouging, underlined by greed and apparent disinterest in the common good. Not to hammer home the point, but Martin Shkreli and the price hike of Daraprim painted a picture of greedy pharmaceutical manufacturers, at least from the point of view of the general public.

There are good reasons for these assumptions that Big Pharma cares only about the bottom line and little about society as a whole. Companies involved with drugmaking often earn billions of dollars a year, and their tendency to raise prices, block patent expirations, and control generic production positions them as the bad guys whose intent is nothing more than price gouging and padding profits while others are forced to spend even higher amounts to obtain drugs. Given all of this, it's easy to put pharmaceutical companies at the center of high drug prices.

So why do these pharmaceutical manufacturers charge so much? It boils down to research and development, administrative costs, and very simply, because they can.

Research Costs

While it's true that Big Pharma seems to make a habit out of squeezing profits out of its many drugs, there is the other side to consider. For one thing, pharmaceutical companies take on high risks, high costs, and low output when they begin working on newer drugs. Getting a drug from concept to market isn't easy; it represents more of a marathon than a sprint. Furthermore, the odds of having a drug approved for sale by the FDA varies from approximately 24 percent (for systemic, anti-infective drugs) to less than 10 percent (for drugs that might be issued to treat cardiovascular, gastrointestinal, or metabolic disorders) (van der Gronde, Uyl-de Groot, and Pieters, 2017). So in a sense, these companies require a great many years and a large capital expense before a drug can even be brought to market, assuming, of course, it is approved for distribution. This is a high-stakes game.

Furthermore, on average, it can take companies ten years to register, test, and release a particular drug, while involving capital investments estimated between $60 million to $2.6 billion. This is a large investment—not to mention a long period of investment in time—for a product that might or might not make it to market.

There is no doubt that drugmaking is a high-risk, high-cost industry. Drug manufacturers also argue the following when it comes to their justified high prices (Kantarjian, Steensma, Sanjuan, Elshaug, and Light, 2014):

- While it's expensive to bring a drug to market, prices are based on the benefit to the patient. The more benefit a drug has to a patient, the higher the cost.
- Free-market forces would eventually bring prices down to reasonable levels.
- Controlling drug prices or increasing price-lowering competition could stifle innovation.

There are, however, fallacies to the above arguments. First, note that the cost of drug development is "much less than commonly reported, as low as 10 percent of the cited $1 billion-plus figure" (p. e208). Furthermore, a cost-benefit analysis doesn't prove any correlation between the price of a drug (specifically, a cancer drug) and objective measures of patient outcomes, such as quality of life or even survival (Kantarjian, Steensma, Sanjuan, Elshaug, and Light, 2014). Finally, the authors point out that lack of market forces available that could drive patented drug prices to reasonable levels, "only what appears to be monopoly pricing" (p. e208).

Other experts cry foul when it comes to linking the ever-increasing prices of drugs with research and development costs (Emanuel, 2019). One study comparing the prices of twenty best-selling drugs in the United States, Europe, and Canada revealed that the cumulative revenue from those drugs more than covered all the drug research and development costs conducted by the fifteen drug companies manufacturing the products (Yu, Helms, and Bach, 2017). Furthermore, after accounting for the $80 billion a year in research, drug companies had $40 billion more from those top twenty drugs alone, all of which went to profits, not research (Emanuel, 2019). Additional profits came from the next one hundred and two hundred brand-name drugs. "We found that premiums pharmaceutical companies earn from charging substantially higher prices for their medications in the US compared to other Western countries, generates substantially more than the companies spend globally on their research and development," the researchers indicated.

It's also difficult to support or refute the drug-research argument as a cost because no one really knows what it actually costs drug companies to conduct research required to obtain FDA approval to bring a product to market (Emanuel, 2019). The best guess came from 2016 report indicating that the cost of bringing a drug to market is $2.6 billion (DiMasi, Grabowski and Hansen, 2016). However, it's difficult to verify the number. The report was produced and released by the Tufts Center, from which more than a quarter of its budget comes from unrestricted grants from pharmaceutical companies and their partners (Emanuel, 2019). It's possible the costs could be lower or higher, though other studies indicate that true drug research dollars can be measured in the millions rather than billions.

What also brings question marks to the research-and-development-expense claim is that pharmaceutical executives themselves acknowledge that overall research activities and similar functions don't determine drug prices. Hank McKinnell, a past CEO of Pfizer, indicated that the primary determinant of price involves "income stream, rather than repayment of sunk costs." Specifically, the estimates of income generated by the sales of medications versus recouping research costs are the reasons for high drug prices (McKinnell and Kador, 2005).

So while there is some merit in pegging research and development as a reason for high drug costs, the argument is somewhat disingenuous.

Getting the Word Out

Another pharmaceutical expense that has been the target of the outrage is promotion, specifically, direct-to-consumer advertising.

Anyone tuning into late-night television will find drug ads promising to cure everything from psoriasis and psoriatic arthritis to inflammation, blood pressure, cholesterol, and so on. There is a reason for all of the ads. Pharmaceutical manufacturers spend a great deal of money on marketing their products.

In 2016, the industry spent $6.1 billion on direct-to-consumer advertising and potentially more than five times as much on marketing to physicians and health care providers (Sarpatwari, DeBello, Zakarian, Najafzadeh, and Kesselheim, 2019).

Most drug advertising takes place on television, in which pharmaceuticals represent the third-highest category of advertising expenditures in 2014, behind automotive and fast-food restaurant advertising (Alpert, Lakdawalla, and Snood, 2015). Nielsen estimated that an average of eighty pharmaceutical ads air every hour on televisions across the US.

So do these tactics work? Are people that gullible that they might be swayed by happy-seeming individuals and peppy music on television? The answer, sadly, is yes. While such promotions do help boost patient awareness of particular drugs and treatments, research shows that marketing also supports overuse of expensive, branded drugs. According to Dee Mangin, associate professor at the Christchurch School of Medicine and Health Sciences in New Zealand (the only other country permitting 100 percent direct-to-consumer advertising of pharmaceuticals), "The truth is, direct-to-consumer advertising is used to drive choice, rather than inform it" (WHO, 2009). There is likely good reason for this. Someone seeing an ad that will cure their feelings of sadness might go to the doctor and beg for the prescription he or she saw on television. And the physician, for other reasons we'll go into later on, will willingly sign that prescription. Hence, advertising can work in this situation.

It's important to understand that direct-to-consumer (DTC) of drugs isn't really new; it has been legal in the United States since 1985 (WHO, 2009). Furthermore, the drug industry has a long history of promoting to the public. Just take a look at any newspaper during the turn of the twentieth century to see all kinds of ads for everything from cocaine drops to elixirs geared to treat nervousness and insomnia.

Drug advertising, as we know it today, took off in 1997 when the FDA eased up on rules requiring drug companies to provide a detailed list of side effects in their television and infomercial advertising.

Overall, marketing by pharmaceutical companies does contribute to higher prescription drug prices in two ways. The first is that such marketing increases prescription drug use (Alpert, Lakdawalla, and Snood, 2015). And second, costs of marketing are part of the overall cost structure of drug manufacturers and put upward pressure on prices (Augustine, Madhavan, and Nass, 2018).

The difficulty in this analysis, however, is that, once again the exact amount that the pharmaceutical industry spends on product promotion is a secret. Much like the costs involved with research and development, no one really knows the true costs of advertising and promotion. According to Alpert et al. (2015), direct-to-consumer advertising of prescription drugs in the United States did increase from $150 million in 1993 to more than $4 billion in 2010. But we really don't know.

Finally, there is the fact that minor improvements in prescription drugs are heralded as major breakthroughs, meaning health care providers are more likely to select the more expensive option, believing that it is the better one (Kantarjian, Steensma, Sanjuan, Elshaug, and Light, 2014). The end result is yet more advertising touting more benefits from the supposedly "new and improved" pharmaceutical product.

The Real Reason for Higher Prices

The main reason why pharmaceutical companies charge higher prices is very simply because they can. Aside from public outrage and the occasional senate hearing or governmental inquiry, nothing changes. Furthermore, thanks to a variety of factors, these pharmaceutical companies are able to operate in an atmosphere of monopoly pricing that is aided and abetted by the US government (Emanuel, 2019). I'll detail this particular issue later on in this book, but the simple explanation is that patent protection, combined with FDA exclusivity, means the US government has granted pharmaceutical companies a monopoly on brand-name drugs. Monopolies mean higher prices, and higher prices will continue until profits fall. Furthermore, the manufacturers do a great job finding loopholes in patent law, meaning that they can continue protecting their high-price products from competition for years, if not decades.

There is little doubt that the pharmaceutical manufacturers must shoulder a great deal of the blame for higher prices. And if this were the only reason for those prices, it would likely be a simple matter to take steps to control such prices, at least from the manufacturing perspective.

But given the current setup, while Big Pharma is a huge cause of skyrocketing drug prices, it is not, by far, the only reason behind it. Other factors, listed below, contribute to the issue as well.

◆ Pharmacy Benefit Managers

Pharmacy benefit managers (PBMs) are the organizations that ostensibly add value and reduce drug costs by managing the pharmaceutical benefits on behalf of an insurance company or plan's sponsor (Drettwan and Kjos, 2019).

PBMs first emerged in the late 1980s as a way to keep rapidly increasing drug prices in check (Dwyer, 2015). Before these benefit managers came on the scene, there was no middleman or structure in place to hold pharmaceutical manufacturers to consistent pricing standards or to guarantee reliable prices from region to region. PMBs worked on this by creating pharmacy networks and offering rebates from pharmaceutical manufacturer. By somewhat "centralizing" the process through linking of the distribution channel (i.e., the pharmacies), it was felt that prices could be better capped.

It isn't really certain, however, that this strategy has been all that effective. These days, the PBMs do more than bring pharmacies and mail-order pharmacies under a network umbrella or offer rebates. The PBMs are the so-called go-betweens that negotiate with drug manufacturers on what medications should be allowed on insurance plans' lists of covered drugs and how much those plans might be willing pay for them—or not (Bluth, 2019). Also negotiated are the rebates a pharma manufacturer pays to the PBM for coverage inclusion on a certain plan. While rebates might mean a drug is covered on a particular insurance plan, more often than not, those savings rarely make it to the consumer (Bluth, 2019).

Here is how it works. Drug manufacturers pay rebates to PBMs after the point of sale; the rebates can make up 40 percent or more of the drug's list price (Seeley and Kesselheim, 2019). PBMs are then reimbursed partially on the rebates they obtain, which are calculated as a percentage of a drug's list price. What this means is that drug manufacturers are, in a sense, paying PBMs to ensure coverage on health care plans in what they call "discounts." And yes, if it might seem as if these rebates, or "discounts," are actually kickbacks, this wouldn't be too far off.

In fact, in most other industries, such a rebate structure could be considered highly illegal due to the kickback components to manufacturers (Gill, 2020). However, one thing that will become evident through this paper is that the pharmaceutical industry is able to operate under rules that are different from other industries. During the early 1990s, the US Department of Health and Human Services (HHS), with backing from Congress, wrote an exception for these payments to federal antikickback laws. This in turn allowed drug companies to use these payments as part of its negotiating toolkit.

The issue with rebating, however, is that the levels are confidential and secret, with the actual cost savings unknown (Drettwan and Kjos, 2019). There is some evidence to suggest that PBMs will sometimes put higher-priced pharmaceuticals as the preferred status on formularies, meaning patients could spend more than they might for lower-cost alternatives that would be equally as effective as their higher-priced counterparts (Seeley and Kesselheim, 2019).

While rebates are suspicious enough, this isn't the sole problem with PBMs. It is that the PBM system pushes a drug's "list" price higher, especially as drug companies continue to find financial wiggle room to provide larger rebates to the PBMs (Gill, 2020). The more the drug companies pay to the PBMs through rebates or discounting, the higher the prices they end up charging. As such, when pharmaceutical manufacturers point fingers, blaming the PBMs for the higher prices they feel they must charge, they aren't too far off. The problem ends up being, however, that while the rebate system might keep some overall costs in check, this can be at the expense of individual patients who require expensive drugs for which there are no substitutes or generic equivalents.

PBMs aren't incentivized to negotiate for lower list prices (Entis, 2019). Rather, their focus is on higher rates because the share of those refunds is how they make their money. Manufacturers, understanding that PBMs want those rebates, have two options. They can either offer a larger discount and earn less money on the drug or offer a larger discount while also increasing the price of the drug. Needless to say, manufacturers will, more often than not, take the latter solution.

PBMs handle other aspects of drug purchasing as well. For instance, when a consumer uses health insurance coverage to fill a prescription, it is the PBM that pays the claim and sets the amount owed by the consumer (Bluth, 2019). This pricing is not the purview of the insurance plan. PBMs also contract with state Medicaid departments and commercial health plans to provide drug coverage for employer-sponsored plans and Medicare Part D enrollees.

PBMs also have power over exclusion lists that specify noncoverage of certain medications, specifically prescription medications that are excluded from insurance coverage. As an aside, it's been noticed that exclusion lists have been growing longer, especially for new, or more expensive, prescription medications (Drettwan and Kjos, 2019).

And as is the case of many activities involving the pharmaceutical industry, PBMs operate secretly, meaning no one can really put a dollar price on what is going on. Much of this is done in secrecy. One such tool that has been used to keep pricing opaque has been gag clauses. Gag clauses are contracts between PBMs and pharmacies, prohibiting the latter from informing a patient as to whether a prescription has alternative purchasing options. The gag clause has recently been legislated out of action, but the onus is now on consumers to ask pharmacies about cheaper drugs.

Adding to the power of PBMs when it comes to pricing and lists is industry consolidation over the past several years (Gill, 2020). Just three PBMs dominate these days. CVS Caremark, Express Scripts, and OptumRX cover more than 150 million individuals, allowing PBMs to be more aggressive when it comes to negotiating with drug manufacturers.

Rebating and other PBM practices have been under public scrutiny as the US grapples with solutions to the high costs of pharmaceuticals. Other PBM-raising red flags include exclusion lists, gag clauses, fluctuations in pharmacy reimbursement rates, and market consolidation.

As such, the question raised is whether PBMs have actually been responsible for a form of price-shifting between stakeholders, meaning an increased profit for themselves and manufacturers and reduced revenues for pharmacies. Furthermore, while some patients and plan sponsors might experience reduced drug prices, this increases prices for other plan sponsors and patients (Lyles, 2017).

Because of the rather tense relationship between pharmaceutical manufacturers and pharmacy benefit managers, it's probably not surprising that both are blaming the others for higher prices (Bluth, 2019). The truth is they are both at fault. But there are other players at work as well.

◆ Health Insurance Companies

While PBMs do set prices and lists for private insurance companies, it is the insurance companies, such as private third-party payers, that must also share some of the blame for higher pharmaceutical costs. Many private insurance companies continue to pass the expense of prescription drugs to their members (in other words, patients and consumers). As more expensive drugs have been coming on the market, and as the prices of most drugs continues increasing, insurers have come up with new ways to require patients to pay a larger share of the cost through coinsurance and higher deductibles and copays. This is known as cosharing of costs, and it ends up costing consumers a lot more money that it did in the past.

Some consumers might be required to copay for a particular drug (along with a deductible or other out-of-pocket costs). Other plans might operate differently. Instead of a flat copay for pharmaceuticals, a consumer's cost for drugs can be calculated as a percentage of the drug's full price, depending on the plan. Note that this percentage is calculated on the drug's full price, *not* the discounted price that the PBM might negotiate for the insurers. Those discounts are not passed down to the consumer, though some insurance companies are rethinking this stance as prices of certain drugs continue to skyrocket.

About one-third to one half of people in commercial plans these days are charged using a coinsurance percentage for certain drugs; this compares to just 3 percent of people enrolled in such plans in 2004 (Gill, 2020). Depending on the drug, an individual could end up paying hundreds of dollars a month for needed drugs.

Another problem involves high-deductible plans that might offer lower premiums up front but require consumers to pay more out-of-pocket fees before insurance reimbursement kicks in (Gill, 2020). Almost half of Americans under the age of sixty-five with private insurance are in such plans, an increase from the 16 percent reported in 2008, according to data from the Centers for Disease Control and Prevention. While private insurers often will cover drug costs without deductible requirements being met, approximately 44 percent of current private plans require that a patient first meet a deductible (either combined with their medical benefit or a separate drug deductible). Until the deductible is met, consumers often must pay the full cost for the drug, versus a flat copay.

Adding to the problem is that between 2010 and 2015, the average annual deductible for employees with health insurance increased by 67 percent. Boiling this down, if a consumer's plan carries a $10,000 deductible, this means that consumer must pay full price for a drug, at least until meeting that deductible. This is a lot of money, and pharmacies (unlike some health care systems) aren't too flexible when it comes to offering payment installment plans.

Then there are the formularies typically developed by health plans, insurance companies, and pharmacy benefit managers. These formularies are lists of drugs covered by payers, involving different tiers of pricing. Sometimes the brand-name drug will be on a higher tier, meaning it is more money for the consumer. Sometimes a generic will be on a lower tier, meaning little to no cost.

Formularies are ostensibly in place to balance the need to manage costs while providing comprehensive therapeutic coverage (American Academy of Actuaries, 2018). The problem comes, however, when a needed drug doesn't have a lower-tier equivalent, which can be the case with many cancer drugs. Additionally, biologics, consisting of pharmaceuticals derived from living cells, are classified as specialty drugs and come with higher prices than traditional brand and generic medications. This means they're going to cost more for the consumers.

Topping it all off is that there is no one set rule for formularies and their costs. They can vary based on plan, deductibility, and other factors. As such, one drug that might not cost very much on one plan could be quite expensive on another. There is just no way of knowing, and the fragmented nature of both the health care insurance industry and the overall health care industry means that one size won't fit all if this is to be corrected.

◆ Retail Pharmacies

The interesting aspect about the pharmaceutical industry is that it operates within a highly specialized distribution environment. Consumers can't just go to their local corner store to pick up a needed drug. Rather, such drugs must be dispensed by state- and federally licensed pharmacies overseen by state- and federally licensed pharmacists. Many of these pharmacies are parts of stores, also known as retail pharmacies. These are located either in stand-alone stores on street corners or shopping centers and can be found in hospitals and other health care centers. While consumers do have the option of purchasing drugs through mail-order pharmacies (which again, need to be licensed by state and federal entities), many will obtain the pharmaceuticals they need through a retail structure. And it's these pharmacies that also can add to the higher price of prescription drugs.

This is because channel intermediaries, which include direct-to-consumer retailers and mail-order, can mark up drug costs far above an average sales price (Kantarjian, Steensma, Sanjuan, Elshaug, and Light, 2014). In other words, they can add their own percentage markup to any prescription drug coming from a wholesaler or manufacturer. Furthermore, there is little standardization as to pricing process. The costs of drugs can vary widely, depending on location and even by pharmacy. It's not uncommon to find two pharmacies located within one block of each other charging different prices for the same drug.

One study highlighting this problem involved research on twelve common drugs and found that "consumers face a dizzying array of pharmacy options as well as significant price differences" among retail pharmacy outlets (Mathew, Kilpatrick, and Garber, 2019). The study's authors noted that large-chain pharmacies tend to charge higher prices than smaller chains or independent pharmacies, even as they have more leverage in the marketplace.

One such example focused on a thyroid enhancement/replacement medicine Levothyroxine (the generic equivalent of Synthroid), which ranged from $4 to $43.71 at various retail pharmacies. Meanwhile, the brand-name drug, Synthroid, ranged in price from $26.64 to $127, depending on the retail pharmacy, location, and whether that pharmacy was located in an urban, suburban, or rural area.

If such price variations between brand-name drugs weren't enough, differentials between retail pharmacies also apply to generics as well. One study analyzing the eleven generic drugs most prescribed by dermatologists found that, even among generics, drug prices varied widely (Alghanem, Abokwidir, Fleischer, Feldman, and Alghanem, 2017). The researchers found that among patients paying cash for their prescriptions, the percentage difference between pharmacies could be up to 35 percent of the total cumulative price for the eleven drugs.

Rite Aid topped the retail pharmacy list for most-expensive generic, followed by CVS, but the CVS prices also differed from state to state. At the other end of the spectrum, Walmart had the lowest prices nationwide, followed by Walgreens.

While the authors of the study acknowledged that the small sample size and study method had its limitations, "larger prospective study is warranted to address the major differences in the price ranges of prescribed medications, and to bring into question the basis of each pharmacies' pricing methods, along with the role their location plays" (p. 128).

The moral of this story, apparently, is that it pays to shop around when it comes to prescription drugs.

◆ Physicians and Health Care Providers

Let's get back to one argument that pharmaceutical manufacturers like to use, which is that free-market mechanics often step in to determine the prices of drugs. This is patently ridiculous as it isn't consumers who determine what drug they will take—unless they see something on late-night TV and then badger their physician to prescribe the product. Private and government-sponsored insurance companies determine whether a consumer can afford a particular drug, and health care providers determine what drugs will be best for the consumers. These providers are the ones who authorize purchase by writing out prescriptions and handing them to consumers or sending them directly to the retail or mail-order pharmacy.

As such, health care providers share much of the responsibility for higher drug prices as it's up to them to prescribe the product. While there might be some kickbacks when it comes to prescribing a certain drug, "health providers often find themselves as reluctant mediators between patients and high-cost pharmaceuticals" (Drettwan and Kjos). The role of the provider is to prescribe, educate, dispense, and even administrate pharmaceuticals.

But doesn't a free-market stance work for health care providers as much as for consumers? Given that health care providers are the decision makers in this case, won't they automatically select something that meets their patients' needs while being affordable? Not really. For one thing, doctors and other providers don't really consider costs of drugs when prescribing. They really can't, because they don't know how much an insurance plan will cover. And adding to the confusion is that pharmaceutical companies promote heavily and directly to physicians and prescribers. We're talking about more than just the occasional flyer or magazine add too. Pharmaceutical companies spend a great deal of one-on-one time with prescribers, directly and consistently promoting to them (Vallenas, 2020).

These are all legitimate ways to promote a product to a target audience. But pharmaceutical companies go beyond simply buying ad space in a medical trade journal or having their sales reps make in-person calls to doctors.

Pharmaceutical companies have been known to provide "incentives" for health care providers, such as paying for continuing medical education lectures or credits (Vallenas, 2020). They might also reach out to physicians and invite them to positive meetings about a new pharmaceutical or offer tickets to various types of entertainment activities. Such incentives can help sway decision-making toward a more expensive drug.

And there's more. Pharmaceutical companies will also staff speakers bureaus with physicians, sending them out to talk about the positive benefits of a drug (and paying them big bucks to do so). This method lends a touch of authenticity to a particular drug. It's much better to see a fellow physician touting the benefits of a new cholesterol or blood pressure medication than to have to listen to the practiced sales pitch of a pharmaceutical representative.

And doctors earn a great deal of money on the Big Pharma payroll (with no law against them doing so). In 2013, ProPublica announced that, in just four years, one doctor had earned $1 million by giving promotional talks and consulting for drug companies, while twenty-one additional doctors had earned more than $500,000 doing the same (Weber and Ornstein, 2013). Interestingly enough, at the time, the ProPublica authors noted that half of the top earners were psychiatrists, prompting James H. Scully Jr., chief executive of the American Psychiatric Association, to say, "It boggles my mind." Scully went on to say that while paid speaking is legal, what was being done was pure marketing.

Despite ProPublica's article (and despite the "often damning scrutiny from prosecutors and academics"), things hadn't settled down by 2019. ProPublica indicated that doctors were still at it, still delivering paid dinner talks and sponsored speeches. According to ProPublica' research, more than 2,500 physicians had received at least half a million dollars (apiece) from drugmakers and medical device companies since 2013; this didn't include monies for research or royalties from inventions (Ornstein, Weber, and Grochowski, 2019).

And when the evidence was presented to Walid Gellad, an associate professor of medicine and health policy at the University of Pittsburgh, he expressed surprise. "Holy smokes," said Gellad, who leads the Center for Pharmaceutical Policy and Prescribing.

The situation wouldn't be quite so alarming if many of the drugs on the list didn't already have a great deal of competition. In one example, seven of the top twenty drugs examined by ProPublica in 2018 treated diabetes. Furthermore, in most of the drug classes on the list, "there are more than one available drug ... indicated for the same condition, selling for high prices," according to Harvard Medical School Professor Aaron Kesselheim (Ornstein, Weber, and Grochowski, 2019). Kesselheim went on to say that "promotional spending is a major way that manufacturers in these situations distinguish themselves from each other—not by conducting comparative studies or by engaging in substantial price reductions." While at one time drug manufacturers extolled their competitive advantage through research abilities, these days, it is how heavily they can promote to doctors.

One example of pharma manufacturers guilty of this type of behavior includes Johnson & Johnson and Bayer AG, manufacturers of blood thinner Xarelto. This drug topped the list in doctor promotional spending from 2014 to 2018, totaling more than $123 million in payments.

This is not to suggest that promotion overall is wrong. Word-of-mouth advertising and testimonials are used frequently in all types of advertising. Testimonials are also important in advertising; they lend a "street cred" to products that might otherwise be lacking. But we aren't talking about a car, piece of furniture, or appliance. We're talking about drugs that affect people's health. As such, the problem here is that promotions of pharmaceuticals encourage physicians to prescribe medications in ways that might not be consistent with evidenced-based practice, while leading to excessive health care spending. This isn't to suggest that doctors are going to prescribe an incorrect medication to a patient because he or she is incentivized to do so by a pharmaceutical manufacturer. It can mean, however, that the doctor in question might be tempted to direct his or her patient to a higher-priced needed medication as opposed to the less expensive equivalent or generic option.

Furthermore, this trend can also lead to overuse of products in situations in which they are medically recommended, leading to negligible or even poor patient outcomes (Vallenas, 2020).

A common example of this tends to be overuse of antibiotics. It's been known for years that antibiotics tend to be overprescribed, used for common ailments such as colds. Research conducted by North Carolina and Georgia health care experts in the field determined that overuse of antibiotics not only places patients at risk for resistance from bacterial diseases but also escalates health care costs (Schultz, Lowe, Srinavasan, and Pugliese, 2014). This is due, in part, to redundant use—using more than one antibiotic for undefined diseases.

How prevalent is this overuse? Well, according to the CDC, one in three antibiotics is inappropriately prescribed, adding an additional $2 billion in health care costs, which also negatively affects clinical quality (Pearl, 2019; CDC, 2016). One study noted that unnecessary antibiotics are prescribed for viral-caused respiratory infections, such as common colds, sore throats, bronchitis, and sinus and ear infections—problems that don't respond to antibiotics (CDC, 2016). Antibiotics should be used for bacterial infections, not those of viral origin.

Furthermore, other researchers found that costs of redundant treatment (such as use of antibiotics when none are really called for) tops $9.9 million and that reducing the use of redundant drugs could reduce the costs (Schultz, Lowe, Srinavasan, and Pugliese, 2014). And this particular research was conducted among only a handful of hospitals. It would be interesting to see what costs can be reduced if physicians stop automatically prescribing antibiotics for every patient presenting with a sniffle.

But the prize for suspicious promotion and horrible patient outcomes—not to mention a huge rise in drug addictions—goes to Purdue Pharma, the company that manufactures the opioid painkiller OxyContin.

These days, just about everyone has been aware of the over-prescribing of pain pills and resulting addictions. However, when Purdue Pharma released OxyContin on the market in 1996, it was aggressively marketed and highly promoted from day one (Van Zee, 2009). In addition to spearheading an aggressive promotional campaign that encouraged physicians to overprescribe the medication for just about any kind of pain, no matter how small, the company substantially invested in pain societies and encouraged the use of opioids when it came to pain management (Vallenas, 2020; Van Zee, 2009). The company also worked hard to influence doctors' prescribing habits by using data to compile profiles on the highest and lowest prescribers of a particular drug, as well as those who were the least discriminate in terms of what they would prescribe (Van Zee, 2009). This meant physicians were specifically targeted for direct promotion by Purdue simply because they overprescribed in the first place. Such overprescribing has been thought to lead to the current opioid crisis faced today in the United States.

Certainly, this goes into the category of overzealous promotion, and Purdue should be held accountable for the rise in opioid addition (which this company is). However, no one held a gun to physicians' heads to prescribe OxyContin. It's assumed that most physicians should know better. While Purdue is not, by all means, the only example, it is the most egregious with its customer-doctors willingly following suit.

While physicians might not be able to prevent ads or pharma reps from their visits, they can have better recognition as to the impact of pharma promotion on prescribing practices and patient outcomes. They can also be a little more aware and willing to research drugs that are effective rather than to buy into rhetoric. In other words, they can rely on evidenced-based practices rather than tickets to seminars for determining the best drugs for their patients.

So what happens when patients are prescribed these high-price medications? Well, 70 percent of physicians who were surveyed by Think-Health and OptomizeMDs indicated that the high cost of prescribed medications leads to unfilled prescriptions (Morse, 2019). The physicians indicated that, while they understood why patients didn't fill prescriptions, few didn't track when or why patients didn't fill the scripts (Morse, 2019). The double whammy here is that these physicians not only prescribed the higher-cost drugs, but they also didn't bother to follow up to ensure compliance or to determine reasons for nonadherence.

In this same survey, the vast majority of patients regularly raised the issue of prescription prices with their doctors, with 86 percent of physicians saying they were comfortable discussing these and other health care costs.

The issue here is that health care providers (as well as consumers) end up bearing the cost when prescriptions aren't filled; there is an increased risk of these patients coming to emergency rooms or emergency departments, or of readmission to hospitals, as conditions worsen. Breaking this into dollars, poor medication adherence costs the US health system as much as $528 billion when it comes to possible consequences, illnesses, and death that can result from nonadherence, according to OptimizeRX.

Physicians can help reduce drug costs for patients, with a little more awareness and a little more attention paid to evidence-based practices.

Then again, there are other stakeholders just outside of the pharmaceutical industry chain that also contribute to higher drug prices, though indirectly.

◆ Greater Life Expectancies

People are living longer than they had been. This in turn tends to ramp up costs in health care across the board. In other words, these greater life expectancies aren't just affecting the price of drugs but are also affecting all types of health care services.

A 2017 article in the *New York Times* pointed out that it isn't just overall aging that is leading to a higher cost when it comes to health care or, by definition, higher pharmaceutical costs (Frakt, 2017). Certainly, individuals who live into their eighties, nineties, and even one hundreds have various health care needs that their grandchildren or great-grandchildren don't. What is boosting up the overall health care cost is overall medical technology. Technology change is responsible for at least one-third per capita of overall health care spending growth, even as some of that technology helps people live longer.

Let's put it this way. At the beginning of the twentieth century, life expectancy in the United States was forty-seven years (Ingram, 2015). These days, in the early part of the twenty-first century, with help from medical technologies, better nutrition, sanitation, and other factors, the US life expectancy is around eighty years old. Much of that is due to more sophisticated health care treatments; fewer children these days are likely to die from whooping cough or measles while older people can go through heart attacks or kidney disease and still have many good years left ahead of them. This was not the case in the early twentieth century.

Speaking of measles and whooping cough, one good example of how medications are prolonging life can be found in vaccinations. Before entering school, for example, children are required to have a series of vaccinations against measles, mumps, and whooping cough, among others. These diseases were once fatal, causing death among much of the younger population. Furthermore, poliomyelitis was once considered a death sentence. Even those who survived might be marred for life, paralyzed and unable to walk. The polio vaccine changed that.

More recently, in the late 1970s and early 1980s, diagnoses of HIV/AIDs or hepatitis C were considered death sentences. However, by 2015, the AIDS mortality rate dropped by 85 percent to fewer than 7,000 deaths a year, from its previous total of 44,000. Meanwhile, hepatitis C cure rates have reached 95 percent. This is all due to research and development of various pharmaceuticals. These drugs have led to prolonging of life.

But sometimes this longevity and survival comes at a cost. One study pointed out that nine out of ten of more than half a million Americans who took at least $50,000 drugs in 2014 were taking so-called "specialty medications" (Swanson, 2015). These are medications that treat both complex and chronic conditions ranging from HIV, AIDs, and cancer to hypertension, rheumatoid arthritis, and kidney failure. These drugs come courtesy of pharmaceutical innovation, which in turn creates means by which people can live longer, healthier lives. However, it also means that the numbers of people on these high-cost drugs are increasing.

Here's the irony. Many of today's pharmaceuticals are geared to help people live longer (or at least more comfortably) by curing or preventing the progression of what were once fatal diseases. But access to pharmaceuticals is increasing the cost of a longer life span, which, in turn, affects older people. This state of affairs will likely continue. And as will be pointed out later on in this paper, older people are at risk from higher costs of pharmaceuticals.

◆ Legislation and Regulation

Before the early 1960s, very few federal regulations existed in the United States when it came to monitoring new drug testing or clinical trials (Tantibanchachai, 2014). Certainly, there was the Pure Food and Drug Act of 1906, but this involved limited legislative oversight. And the original Food, Drug and Cosmetic Act of 1938 required that a new drug had to be safe. But "safe" could mean a variety of things.

All things considered, no specific laws required physicians to keep logs of prescribed drugs, nor were the doctors required to follow up with their patients.

Then thalidomide came along.

First developed by Swiss pharmaceutical company CIBA in the early 1950s, thalidomide was sold in Germany by Chemi Grunenthal under the brand name of Contergan (Bennett, 2020). The drug, first introduced as a sedative, had undergone only basic testing, which determined it wouldn't have toxic effects on humans.

Meanwhile, in Europe, the drug was receiving rave reviews. Thalidomide was considered a miracle cure, with some claiming it could treat everything from macular generation to diabetes, auto-immune diseases, and cancer (Tantibanchachai, 2014). By the late 1950s, thalidomide was marketed in forty-six countries. As time went on, thalidomide became popular as a remedy for morning sickness among pregnant women, made more appealing by the fact that it could be obtained without a prescription.

This great news made its way to the United States where the extensive testing of new drugs was not as stringent as it is today. In 1960, US company Richardson-Merrell decided to sell thalidomide, under the brand name of Kevadon (Tantibanchachai, 2014). The corporation applied to the FDA, asking for approval to sell the drug as a treatment for a variety of ailments, including morning sickness among pregnant women. Yet all was not right with thalidomide. FDA physician and pharmacist Frances Kelsey was leery of the drug, reading about studies demonstrating adverse complications of the drug, including birth defects. She requested more information from Richardson-Merrell about thalidomide's impact, especially on pregnant women.

At the same time, Tennessee Senator Estest Kefauver was also investigating the drug, basing it on his desire to introduce a bill enhancing safety regulations of drugs.

There were good reasons for Kefauver's and Kelsey's concerns, namely because of reports from Japan, Australia, and Europe indicating a link between pregnant mothers who had taken thalidomide for morning sickness and gave birth to offspring with congenital mutations (Bennett, 2020). Other problems reported included eye problems, facial palsies, internal organ damage, and ear disfigurement.

It's important to point out that thalidomide was never formally approved for use in the United States. It didn't undergo massive drug trials, but its properties for cures were assumed. And assuming the drug would receive FDA acceptance, Richardson-Merrell had already distributed more than 2.5 million thalidomide tablets to approximately 1,200 physicians. These doctors, in turn, gave the tablets to 20,000 patients in clinical trials; at least 207 of whom were pregnant at the time. Among the pregnant women, seventeen reported birth defects among their infants. Furthermore, there were no records kept as to who was given the drug. Richardson-Merrell gave the drug to the physicians, who gave them to patients, and left it at that. There were no stringent requirements involved with this, which was another tragedy involving this drug.

The reason why the thalidomide story is so important is because it ultimately led to the 1962 Kefauver-Harris Amendments to the Food, Drug, and Cosmetic Act. It also led to Frances Kelsey's status of hero for preventing a potentially dangerous drug (at the time) from receiving FDA approval.

Meanwhile, the Kefauver-Harris Amendments, which went into effect in 1963, required that drug manufacturers prove the effectiveness of drug products before going on the market and to report serious side effects (FDA, 2012). Other requirements of the amendments include that (FDA, 2012)

- evidence of effectiveness be based on well-controlled clinical studies, conducted by qualified experts
- study subjects provide informed consent
- the FDA be given 180 days to approve a new drug application, with FDA approval required before the drug is marketed in the United States

- the FDA have regular inspection of production facilities
- the FDA have control of pharmaceutical advertising, including listing of drug side effects

Interestingly enough, thalidomide is in use today as a treatment for multiple myeloma and leprosy (Bennett, 2020). The difference, of course, is that this drug's reintroduction underwent a series of research and clinical trials to determine safety and efficacy. Additionally, side effects of the drug are generally known, which they weren't in the late 1950s and early 1960s.

There is some irony to the Kefauver-Harris Amendments—namely that one reason why Senator Kefauver introduced the bill in the first place was due to excessive drug prices (Greene and Podolsky, 2012). Furthermore, no one is denying that drugs should be tested for efficacy and potential side effects (with those side effects clearly delineated) before coming to market.

However, the burden of proof required to ensure safety and efficacy of drugs has meant the process of developing pharmaceuticals became longer and more expensive (Greene and Podolsky, 2012). This in turn created what was known as "drug lag," in which innovative compounds came to Europe long before they were available on the US market. This difficulty, in turn, led to modification in the Drug Price Competition and Patent Term Restoration Act of 1984, which further extended drug patents.

Another unintended consequence of Kefauver-Harris was that structures of proof changed conceptual categories relied on by international biomedical researchers. Specifically, pharmaceutical research became organized around the placebo-controlled, randomized trial to ensure efficacy of the products. While this system has helped gauge the potency and effectiveness of individual drugs, it also means data on comparative efficacy more difficult and more expensive to find and produce. It simply takes longer to get drugs from the concept/need to completion, or the market.

Boiling all of this down, increased regulation and legislation has added costs to drug research, development, and manufacturing—costs that are passed down to insurance companies and consumers. As such, "the Kefauver's amendments ultimately affected both pharmaceutical pricing and patenting—in a manner diametrically opposed to the one (Kefauver) intended." In this case, Big Pharma does have it right. Drug costs are huge, and partly because of the required testing before release.

None of this suggests that drugs shouldn't be carefully tested before being released to the public. The last thing we need, as a society, are poor side effects from drugs such as thalidomide. The truth, however, is that because drug development is highly regulated, the research and development process is longer. This leads to more drug dropouts during a drug's development process, which increases invested time and costs in research (van der Gronde, Uyl-de Groot, and Pieters, 2017).

In addition to tacking on more costs to drugs, this leads to high barriers to entry in the industry. It requires a great deal of capital to go up against Big Pharma's "big guns," not to mention the sheer amount of resources required to get a drug researched, tested, and manufactured. This makes it difficult for smaller companies to register drugs, which limits the number of firms that have enough resources to invest in drug research. Lack of competition leads, once again, to monopolistic pricing.

Then there is the approval process itself, overseen by the US Food and Drug Administration. The FDA requires a great deal of data before it will OK a drug for sale, which is not the problem. The problem is that approval of pharmaceuticals in the United States has little to do with pricing or cost effectiveness. Regulatory agencies allow drugs to be released to the market based on safety and effectivity, but not with reference to either price or cost effectiveness. This means the price and reimbursement of a drug are determined only after registration approval and insurance company or government negotiation. It also paves the way for very high-priced drugs, which would include biologics and to an extent genetic drugs, which are just starting to come onto the market.

Additionally, the FDA doesn't consider pricing—or competition—during the drug's approval process. As long as a drug is proven to be safe for human use, and is effective, it can be approved, even if a more cost-effective solution exists (Alvaro, Challener, and Branch, 2019). This lack of accountability encourages pharmaceutical manufacturers to come out with a lot of the same drug simply to make more money rather than to actually put medications on the market. This is why, for example, there are several different types of insulin on the market (and no generic equivalent, interestingly enough). These different types of insulin basically do the same thing, but because there is a lot money in treating diabetes, there is more insulin. The price doesn't go down because of competition, however. Due to minute molecular changes between brands, different patents have been issued for different types of insulin, meaning monopolistic pricing practices are in play.

This is also the reason why there are four erectile dysfunction drugs on the market these days (not to mention a "daily" version) (Harvard Health Publishing, 2020). There really is no need for this much medication for what is really not a fatal medical problem. However, there is good money to be made in drugs that massage the male ego, so to speak. The FDA doesn't care; its concern is safety and efficacy. So we now have four similar drugs on the market, to treat one condition that is questionable as a health issue. Simply because it produces revenue. Perhaps on the positive side, there are generic equivalents. But the issue here is that there really isn't the need for this much in the first place.

Can't legislators—or the FDA—do anything about this state of the affairs? Well, yes. But Big Pharma has been able to strike fear into the hearts of legislators whenever discussion about curbing prices comes up in discussion. The main argument of pharmaceutical manufacturers—that higher prices are justified due to research and development, and curbing prices will, in turn, curb innovation—has a dire impact on those who develop and enforce policy. Noted Ezekiel Emanuel (2019),

> Every time Congress debates doing something about drug prices, the industry … vociferously returns to the point that lower prices will thwart innovative research. The fear if missing a cure for Alzheimer's or Lou Gehrig's disease or depression contributes to stalling reform.

In other words, for all the posturing and complaints about higher prices from Congress, the FDA, and even the president of the United States, don't expect much to be done form a legislative standpoint.

◆ Additional Causes

The above makes it very clear that the high drug prices can be based on more than one cause. But there are other factors that also lead to a markup in these prices, which need to be noted for complete understanding as to why it's so difficult to get control over what is happening. Some of these reasons are listed below.

Overutilization

In addition to changes in disease prevalence and more effective disease identification (meaning more drug use), overutilization is a concern. Pharmacies, for example, are reimbursed by the number and day supply of prescriptions they fill, while pharmaceutical manufacturers receive income based on volume of pharmaceuticals that is driven off formulary placement (American Academy of Actuaries, 2018). Direct-to-consumer marketing can also lead to overutilization. As mentioned earlier, such advertising and promotion creates demand from patients who observe drug advertisements for a particular condition they might have then request that their physicians prescribe those drugs without appropriate information on alternatives or side effects (American Academy of Actuaries, 2018).

Cost per Unit

Brand-name drugs typically experience higher price increases as their exclusivity periods come to an end (American Academy of Actuaries, 2018). This is vastly different from lifecycles of other products. The longer they are on the market, the more "mature" they become, meaning price drops. Not so with prescription drugs. New brand drugs are often introduced to the market at higher prices than the current drugs they are meant to replace (American Academy of Actuaries, 2018). Switching to generic drugs, in the past, has typically resulted in lower prices. However, some new generics have come with high unit costs, while other generics have experienced substantial price increases, due to acquisitions or repricing (American Academy of Actuaries, 2018).

Specialty Drugs

Specialty drugs are pharmaceuticals that are considered high cost and/or high complexity. By their nature, these specialty drugs are driving up costs of pharmaceuticals overall. The other viewpoint, however, is that as high as the costs of these specialty products are, they could also help avoid more expensive medical procedures down the road. One such example is the previously mentioned example is Sovaldi, introduced by Gilead Sciences to treat hepatitis C (American Academy of Actuaries, 2018). It was released in late 2013, at a price of $84,000 for the twelve-week treatment (American Academy of Actuaries, 2018).

While this treatment is extremely costly, the question is whether untreated hep C might end up being even more expensive; left untreated, this disease could lead to liver cancer or the need for a liver transplant. A liver transplant is generally more expensive than the drugs, not to mention potentially leading to increased trauma and future complications and health risks to the patient. It's also true that not all individuals with untreated hep C will require transplants. It's an either-or scenario. Both options are hugely expensive. But the question boils down to which option will end up being more expensive in the long run. With this in mind, Solvadi is cheaper than a hospital stay or liver transplant.

Lack of Central Negotiating Authority

This is a huge issue, and one of the main reasons why drug prices are so confusing (as well as being so high). The United States is the only industrialized nation that lacks any kind of central group or committee that has as its sole charge negotiating for reasonable drug prices. In Canada and many European nations, the government takes responsibility for negotiating with pharmaceutical companies. In the US, however, the federal government is actively prohibited from negotiating prices for populations other than Medicaid beneficiaries and military veterans. This means commercial populations are subsidizing low costs in these negotiated areas. The federal government can't even negotiate directly with manufacturers for Medicare beneficiaries, thanks to the Medicare Improvement Act of 2003 and the rise of Medicare Part D. Part D program beneficiaries—age sixty-five plus—are among the largest users of medications.

Along these lines, the US drug market is highly fragmented, another factor contributing to the higher prices (Alvaro, Challener, and Branch, 2019). Because no universal or singular regulatory agency negotiates drug prices, insurance companies find themselves in the position of dealing directly with the pharmaceutical manufacturers.

Different insurance companies differ, leading to less leverage and buying power as a whole, and higher cost. These are then shifted to the consumer.

Medicare Part D Protected Class

Finally, there is the issue of the so-called "protected" class of drugs under Medicare Part D. These drugs and therapies are "protected," because they can't be dropped from the Medicare Part D list. The original idea of "protected classes" was proposed in 2005, before the program's official launch. (Interestingly enough, it wasn't included as part of the Medicare Improvement Act.) The protected class policy was introduced out of concerns that transition to Medicare drug coverage might disrupt continuous coverage of needed drugs for certain conditions and beneficiaries, who might otherwise have been discouraged from enrollment in Part D (Kocot, McCutcheon, and White, 2019).

With help from subregulatory guidance, the Centers for Medicare and Medicaid (CMS) directed the Part D sponsors to initially include "all or substantially all" drugs in six categories for coverage on all Part D formularies (Kocot, McCutcheon, and White, 2019). These were antidepressants, antipsychotics, immunosuppressants, antiretrovirals, and antineoplastics.

The protected class guidance was meant to be short term; it was in place during the first-year transition to Part D coverage, allowing full access to all drugs in these classes for vulnerable Part D beneficiaries. It remains in place because of concerns over protection of certain drugs. The concerns, rightfully so, center around a needed drug that might be inadvertently struck off the list, which could be problematic for a consumer who relies on that particular drug.

The problem, however, is that the term "protected classes" means that lack of competition has provided the motivation to increase drug prices on the part of the manufacturers. The pharma makers understand that their drugs can't be removed from the list due to higher prices. These pharmaceuticals, after all, are "protected" and must remain. And once again, Medicare is prohibited, by law, from renegotiating many of these drug prices (Khullar and Bach, 2020). The protected class add-on, meant to be only temporary and meant to help ensure that beneficiaries were provided for, has become a costly "extra," despite the attempts of two presidential administrations to change it.

◆ The "Single-Source" Fallacy

Specifically, the complex nature of the overall health care system—involving patients, clinicians, hospitals, insurance companies, drug companies, pharmacists, pharmacy benefit managers, and government organizations—makes it extremely difficult to put into place one single policy or solution to reduce drug prices (Augustine, Madhavan, and Nass, 2018). This complexity makes it enormously difficult to understand the factors contributing to drug costs. Added to the scenario is that little public information is available concerning financial transactions between various participants in the pharmaceutical supply chain.

This is why, for instance, as well-meaning as the Trump administration's efforts to lower drug prescriptions are, they don't do much to attack the many root problems. Executive orders are all well and good, but they don't do much to target the entire industry and the problem with pricing. Later in this paper, we'll examine both President Trump's executive orders and President-Elect Joe Biden's proposed policies toward reducing drug prices. Suffice it to say, however, that the solution—or rather solutions—will need to involve more than political policies or executive orders.

BIG PHARMA: AN ECONOMICS OVERVIEW

TO TRULY UNDERSTAND THE PROBLEM OF DRUG PRICING requires an economic discussion about the pharmaceutical industry and how it operates. As we saw above, the fault of high drug prices doesn't belong to any one entity or factor. Rather, the ever-continuing higher prices are the result of the influence of a complex and highly interactive set of factors and can be summed up by the following:

- high launch prices with the price of the drug often increasing over time
- lack of competition when market exclusivity ends
- lack of effective incentives for controlling the product's price
- unequal bargaining power between buyers and sellers
- research, development, marketing, and administrative expenditures
- the design of insurance programs, including patient cost-sharing provisions

- poor performance of patient assistance programs and other public programs in place to help make medicines more affordable
- lack of adequate information in place to help drive choices regarding medications

This section will allow a more careful look at the economics of pharmaceuticals and the determination of how those economics end up with higher prices.

One driver of continued skyrocketing drug prices can be put to the nature of the pharmaceutical industry itself. While Big Pharma and others consistently point out that capitalization is OK, and there is plenty of competition between different companies and manufacturers, in truth, this industry doesn't fit anything regarding a capitalistic structure. In fact, van der Gronde et al. (2017) point out that "market failure, in combination with higher merger and acquisition activity in the sector have allowed price increases for even off-patent drugs."

The industry likes to tout itself as an example of a capitalistic free market, which along with supply and demand (not to mention the above-mentioned large costs of development, research, regulations, and bringing a pharmaceutical to market) determines pricing. Because the pharmaceutical industry considers itself "competitive," it can claim that supply and demand (especially demand) determine market price.

This could be accepted if 1) consumers were actually the decision-maker when it comes to buying pharmaceuticals, 2) the decision makers (prescribers) weren't targeted and promoted so hard to influence decision-making that might be in contrast to evidenced-based practice, and 3) the US government wasn't actively creating a monopolistic environment in which pharmaceutical companies are operating. Basically, a truly free and competitive market, one in which pricing is based on that competition, would come without patent regulation, rebates, formularies, or evergreens, all of which are a large part of drug pricing. As such, in free-market economies, most commodities are priced according to what the market will bear. Specifically, this means a price that focuses on an item's scarcity, the utilitarian value of the commodity, demand for the product, and supply (Kantarjian, Steensma, Sanjuan, Elshaug, and Light, 2014). There are comments from pharmaceutical executives that their pricing *is* what the market will bear. This is not really true. Pharmaceuticals follow their own pricing rules that don't have much to do with what the market will bear.

◆ The Decision Makers

Let's take a look at the economics involved with the free-market purchase of an appliance such as a refrigerator. If someone wants to buy a refrigerator, he or she will shop around, compare prices and amenities, and then, if both are agreeable with this individual, buy that product. If a lot of people are attached to that particular fridge, demand will increase and the price will increase. Or the manufacturer of that product will attempt to stimulate demand by lowering the price through some kind of rebate or sale. Once that refrigerator has worn out its welcome on the market—in other words, it costs more to manufacture it than the price that is being paid—it will retire and no more of that particular product will roll off the assembly lines.

One major way in which pharmaceuticals differ from fridges is that the former's sector is extraordinarily complex. It doesn't begin with the consumer. Rather, it begins with a "prescription." In actuality, it begins with what the drugmaker thinks will make the most money. In either case, the consumer is not the driver of this "free market." Both federal and state laws regulate consumer access to certain types of drugs; such approval can only be approved by a health care provider before those drugs are sold to patients. Basically, a consumer can only acquire a prescription from a health care provider who is licensed to practice in the state in which the consumer lives. As such, while the consumer has need of a particular drug, it is the physician, nurse practitioner, or physician's assistant who can authorize the consumer to buy it.

Furthermore, the consumer can't stop off at one of many stores to buy the product in question. Rather, the consumer is allowed to purchase the drug from a government-licensed pharmacy, either retail or mail-order. These distribution points, in turn, have purchased the products from wholesalers who have, in turn, acquired them from the manufacturers. This isn't too far off from the refrigerator example. What really puts the confusion into the whole situation is third-party interference, in the form of health insurance, which adds yet another piece of red tape to the already cluttered decision-making process of the supposed "free market" of pharmaceuticals. Health insurance is either privately run (third party payers supported by employers or, in more recent years, the Affordable Care Act marketplace) or government funded (Medicare and Medicaid).

While the overall health care insurance market is hugely complex, it becomes even more complicated for prescription drugs. Drug insurance plans tend to eliminate any kind of patient price-sensitivity (Ellyson and Basu, 2018).

This is because health insurance plans intervene to pay for drugs, while pharmacy benefit managers, which are intermediaries, interact with the prescription drug insurers to negotiate the prices, both with manufacturers and retail pharmacies. Adding to this, drug manufacturers frequently offer price rebates to PBMs, but no meaningful information exists to determine the actual size of those rebates or how much PBMs retain of those rebates as profit.

Another complexity is that pharmaceutical companies advertise their products directly to consumers, in some cases offering patients copay coupons to offset cost-sharing of payments required by many prescription drug insurance plans. The net effect of this particular model is to steer customers toward selecting the more expensive drug, meaning the insurance company incurs the cost which, in turn, means overall higher premiums.

In a sense, what this means is there is no free-market decision the consumer can make when it comes to determining what prescription drug to buy. Rather, it is the licensed health care provider that determines a need, a specially licensed distribution point that allows the consumer to buy it, and middleman along the distribution chain that determines pricing through confusing and—more often than not—opaque methods that prohibit any kind of meaningful price comparisons between products. Even if a consumer prices a generic medication with its brand-name counterpart, that individual can't buy that product, unless the doctor checks the "substitution OK" box on a prescription. And it's likely that the consumer might not think to ask about it.

Furthermore, because physicians determine what drug is prescribed, they rarely have any direct incentive to select the most cost-effective treatment for a patient (Sarpatwari, DeBello, Zakarian, Najafzadeh, and Kesselheim, 2019). In fact, as mentioned above, they might be incentivized by pharmaceutical manufacturers to steer consumers to more expensive drugs. The exception here is that if the drug in question is a "specialty" drug with no competition—in which case, the pharma manufacturer can price it to whatever level it wants or what the market will bear. This leads to something else—namely that physicians and other health care providers can often be unaware of absolute or relative prices of drugs. This is especially the case of the specialty, or newer, drugs coming to the market.

Finally, the degree to which there is interference along the drug supply chain, patients aren't exposed to the "real" price of pharmaceuticals, so really has no basis of comparison as to whether a particular drug is priced too high or not. As a result, they don't have enough incentive to shop for lower-cost alternatives which, in turn, eliminates any downward pressure on price of new or existing brand-name, or even generic, pharmaceuticals. As a result, "both incumbent drug manufacturers and potential entrants face a pricing decision under which increasing price is the dominant strategy," note Ellyson and Basu (2018, p. 6).

Going even further, the economists suggest that what they call "pipeline pressure" actually drives increases in the price of current drugs as manufacturers continue to hold on to their market share and profits.

The end result of the economic distribution/supply chain of pharmaceuticals is that consumers have absolutely no pricing power. This is also characterized by the following:

- physicians not having the market knowledge or intelligence to prescribe the most cost-effective treatments
- constraints on payers' abilities to compare, or set, one drug manufacturer against another when it comes to drug price negotiations
- misdirected incentives that allow pharmacy benefits managers to accept high-list prices of brand-name drugs

The above is "strike one" when it comes to Big Pharma's— and others'—assertions that pharmaceutical pricing is due to a free-market mechanism. The other issue is that of government interference and its promotion of a monopolistic environment in which Big Pharma can operate.

◆ The Government's Hand

The United States, on the surface, is in a pitched battle against businesses focused on monopolistic practices. The bottom line is that the US government tends, in theory, to take a dim eye to monopolistic competitive practices.

The Sherman Act of 1890, the Clayton Act of 1914, and the Federal Trade Commission Act of 1914 are all geared to ensure that no company can shut out competition or monopolize a product or service. The FTC, in fact, is adamant that monopolization is bad, pointing out that penalties for violating the Sherman Act can be severe, while the FTC itself is in the business of banning "unfair method of competition" (FTC, 2020).

Yet all of the above seems to go out the window when it comes to the pharmaceutical industry. Basically, the government is complicit in providing a perfect environment in which monopolistic practices seem to be encouraged.

Because pharmaceutical companies wouldn't ordinarily be able to profit from new drug development, the US government has stepped in to protect companies in two ways: patent protection and market exclusivity. While both of these tools are similar, they do differ in that they are governed and overseen by different statutes (FDA (c), 2020).

Patents

Patents are a property right that is granted by the United States Patent and Trademark Office and can be filed at any point during a drug's development (FDA (c), 2020). Patents can encompass a wide range of claims (FDA (c), 2020). Furthermore, new patents can be filed if there is some kind of change in the drug; this can be a chemical change or even the shape of the medication itself. Patent terms are set by statute, with the term of a new patent being twenty years from the date on which the patent application was filed in the United States (FDA (c), 2020; van der Gronde, Uyl-de Groot, and Pieters, 2017). Sometimes, a patent can be extended to twenty-five years or longer. Exact timing can be affected by a variety of factors (FDA (b), 2020).

The drug patent system is often blamed for higher prices because it limits competition while creating monopolies. While revising the patent system could prevent abuse (especially as pharmaceutical companies continue seeking to exploit the repatenting loophole), removing that system completely would "significantly reduce companies' incentive to invest in research" (van der Gronde, Uyl-de Groot, and Pieters, 2017, p. 21).

Market Exclusivity

While patents protect formulas, manufacturing processes and other factors related to the drug itself, exclusivity is more focused on delays and prohibitions concerning competitor drugs (FDA (b), 2020). In other words, assuming that the brand-name manufacturer files the correct paperwork, the FDA can prohibit competition from coming into the market and taking potential profits away from the pharmaceutical company (FDA (b), 2020). A new drug application (NDA) or abbreviated new drug application (ANDA) holder is eligible for exclusivity, so long as statutory requirements are met (FDA (b), 2020). Patents can also be granted for new chemical entities, allowing companies to charge higher prices once the drug is ready for marketing.

Much like patents, exclusivity terms can vary; according to the FDA, "it depends on what type of exclusivity is at issue." On average, drug exclusivity is generally granted for approximately seven years for "orphan" drugs and five years for new chemicals, with an additional period of six months of exclusivity following pediatric approval (van der Gronde, Uyl-de Groot, and Pieters, 2017, Ciociola, Cohen, and Kulkarni, 2014).

Breaking this down further, there is a five-year exclusivity for small molecules, a twelve-year exclusivity period for biologics, and six-month pediatric exclusivity (Engelberg, 2015). These and other exclusivities continue to be granted, without regard for the investment required or any value produced (Engelberg, 2015).

In all fairness, one reason for patents and market exclusivity is due to excessive regulation of drugs in the first place. Because it does take a long time to get a drug through research, development, clinical trials, peer-reviewed research, and everything else to market. As such, it isn't fair to subject a brand-new drug that costs who-knows-how-much-money to manufacture, to the rigors of competition. This is, after all, why the patents and exclusivity are in place. Pharmaceutical companies should be able to recoup their costs and earn a nice profit in providing a benefit to society.

While there is no question that brand-name drug companies should be allowed to retain both patent and exclusivity when it comes to earning a profit, it has gone too far as drug companies are using the patent system not to recoup expenses (and then some) from a product but to "avoid competition in order to earn outsized profits on medicines for many years beyond what was intended (I-MAK, 2018). As mentioned above, drug manufacturers can continue filing patents on making tiny changes to existing drugs, thus extending their profits. It's also this type of loophole that allows the Vyera Pharmaceuticals of the world to increase the prices of Daraprim simply because continued patents protect its pricing. This means no competition and no incentive for the company to keep prices low.

In addition to exclusivity and patents, there are two other ways in which government helps set up a monopolistic environment for pharmaceutical manufacturers (Engelberg, 2015). For one thing, federal law actually prohibits the FDA from approving a copy of a new drug for a period from seven to twelve years, even if no patents have been filed. Additionally, the FDA can't approve a generic drug for use, as long as a pharmaceutical manufacturer alleges patent infringement. Needless to say, this has encouraged "many frivolous patent claims, just to delay competition" (Engelberg, 2015).

While the US government likes to regularly remind us that it is supportive of capitalism and disdains monopolistic practices, its behavior in regard to the pharmaceutical industry suggests otherwise. Over the years, both US agencies and Congress have created a web of monopolies, with the result being that the United States is paying the world's highest prices for pharmaceuticals. If the government wants to tackle the high prices of prescription drugs, it should first examine the patents and exclusivity it permits Big Pharma when it comes to manufacturing and pricing these products.

◆ No to Negotiation—or Comparisons

The hallmark of a capitalistic system is the ability of the consumer to compare and contrast pricing and benefits. We saw this in the example of the refrigerator, above. But as has been made fairly clear by now, Big Pharma tends to play by different rules when it comes to much of anything capitalistic, and this includes price matching. This is because industry itself is highly opaque when it comes to pricing strategies. No one really knows how much a drug costs to manufacturer, or even knows the exact "list" price that can be paid. Apparently, this is a large secret. Even worse, the

Patient-Centered Outcomes Research Institute—PCORI—is prevented from determining cost comparisons and cost effectiveness in its recommendations (Kantarjian, Steensma, Sanjuan, Elshaug, and Light, 2014). PCORI is responsible for evaluating treatments for coverage by federal programs. Because PCORI is unable to obtain the information necessary to make the right determinations in terms of medications, it is unable to make valid recommendations to assist both consumers and health care professionals in obtaining the best, cost-effective treatments. It must make those recommendations without the benefits of data, meaning prescribers must authorize medications while crossing their fingers that the medications don't create too much of a price burden on their patients.

Speaking of government agencies, it's been mentioned before, but it bears repeating Medicare has no negotiating power when it comes to dealing with pharmaceutical manufacturers. The misnamed Medicare Reform Act of 2003 put into place legislation prohibiting Medicare from negotiation. Rather, the program is offered through private insurance providers, and it is these providers that must singly go to the pharmaceutical manufacturers and negotiate separately for prices. If Medicare had the power to directly negotiate, it could help reduce drug prices, especially among the elderly, who could certainly use a hand in this scenario. It's estimated that allowing Medicare to negotiate drug prices could save approximately $40 billion to $80 billion per year (Baker, 2006).

However, the lack of an ability to negotiate, in combination with the Medicare expansion in 2006 (which added various and additional prescription drug benefits to the entire package), meant more—and higher—profits to pharmaceutical companies.

◆ Brand-to-Brand Competition: Can It Work?

Let's get back to the refrigerator. Maytag fridges regularly compete against those manufactured by Amana, Westinghouse, Sony, Whirlpool, and LG, and no one bats an eyelid. In fact, it's expected.

Some well-meaning individuals have pointed out that accelerating approval of non-first-in-class drugs to promote brand-to-brand competition could lower prices. Again, in a typical (i.e., nonpharmaceutical) sector, this would work. However, research involving the potential of brand-brand competition noted that few price-lowering controls were in effect when a new drug entry took place, especially among intraclass brand-name drug prices (Sarpatwari, DeBello, Zakarian, Najafzadeh, and Kesselheim, 2019). Anyone comparing the price of the various insulin drugs on the market would likely agree with this result.

One study did, however, indicate that brand-brand competition could anchor list prices of new drugs below what they might be, in the absence of any competition. Furthermore, the effect of brand-brand competition on drug prices could be modified by relative drug quality, with safer and/or more effective new drugs commanding higher prices along with greater marketing, when it comes to higher intraclass prices.

Would it then make sense to boost brand-to-brand competition? Not necessarily, and for the same reason I've been demonstrating all along in this section. It's impossible to compare the pharmaceutical industry to any other one. The overall economic theory when it comes to more products on the market rests on the idea that the higher degree of competition of a good, the lower the demand. This is due to the supply/demand factor, which indicates that the higher the competition, the more goods are available, meaning lower demand and lower prices.

While theoretical economics demonstrates that entry of new products (or even potential entry of new products) tends to drive markets to a more efficient allocation of resources, research also suggests that there are many anticompetitive strategies that a firm can put into place to deter entry of competition (Ellyson and Basu, 2018). The pharmaceutical industry has been a master at employing these strategies. Not that there is price collusion between, say, Pfizer and Eli Lilly (that *would* have the Federal Trade Commission involved). But pharma manufacturers with brand-name drugs already on the market have an incentive to slowly increase prices, retain as much market share as possible, and slow the learning process about new drugs (potentially competitive drugs) entering the market (Ellyson and Basu, 2018; Ching, 2010). We'll delve into this in more detail in the next section covering generic drugs.

◆ No, It's Not "Competitive"

To conclude, there is little that is "competitive" about the pharmaceutical sector, at least from the economic point of view. The pharmaceutical supply chain is not driven by competitive market forces. Rather, it represents the action of profit-seeking firms that are "operating within an extremely complex array of privileges and constraints set by the government." The government interactions include research funding, granting of market exclusivity, enforcing strict product requirements and standards, and even acting as the ultimate buyer for a large swath of the population. "Simply stated, the typical presumption that market forces will work—and work best—does not hold well for the biopharmaceutical sector."

Rather, the pharmaceutical industry is well-entrenched and well-established in monopolistic practices, which have been aided and abetted by the federal government. Until and unless some of these loopholes are found and plugged, and until antitrust laws are taken seriously by the industry, lobbyists, and Congress, any kind of meaningful reform will be very difficult to enact and make stick. As such, while the industry likes to present itself as working in capitalistic confines, it is, in fact, anything but.

THE STORY OF GENERICS

WHEN IT COMES TO THE QUESTION ABOUT HOW TO lower the cost of pharmaceuticals in the United States, the discussion invariably turns to the thought that generic drugs are a tool that could help. Generics, by their nature, mean lower prices. Anyone shopping for a laundry detergent in a store understands that it costs a great deal less than a brand-name counterpart, namely because that brand name automatically carries a price increase.

Generic drugs aren't too different from that detergent. Generics are defined as the "bioequivalent replicas of brand-name drugs, containing the same active ingredients and with identical quality, safety, and efficacy profiles" (Wouters, Kanavos, and McKee, 2017, p. 555). Differences between generic and name-brand drugs are with inactive ingredients, such as coloring, flavoring, and stabilizing ingredients. Generics aren't necessarily new; they've been around for quite a few years. Historically, the United States has had high rates of generic drug use; in 2013, 84 percent of prescriptions were filled using generics. But understanding why generics are not exactly a cure-all when it comes to higher drug prices requires a bit of in-depth analysis.

◆ The Troubled History behind Generics

While (in theory) generic drugs should help reduce overall pharma costs, not every stakeholder involved has supported the idea of such substitutions for use in the marketplace. Over the years, and perhaps unsurprisingly, trade organizations for brand-name drugmakers have consistently and regularly resisted generic drug policy reforms. Generics have "a history marked by political conflicts, vested economic interests, and intense lobbying by stakeholders" (Wouters, Kanavos, and McKee, 2017, p. 574). Put another way, drugmakers don't like generic counterparts because they take away market share and, more importantly, profits.

Such lobbying and antigeneric stances reach back to the mid-twentieth century, during the time when new drugs were being researched and introduced to the market in vast quantities. The first instances of generic drug substitutions took place during the late 1940s, and trade organizations, including the National Pharmaceutical Council (NPC), American Medical Association (AMA) and American Pharmacists Association (AphA) were not at all happy about it. These organizations lobbied vociferously against such substitutions, claiming they would stifle innovation and research while reducing quality of care. These organizations' efforts successfully tapped into fears that generic drugs might not be as effective as their brand-name counterparts. The result was that by 1959, forty-four states had enacted laws preventing generic drug substitutions for the brand-name pharmaceuticals.

This state of affairs lasted until the 1960s and 1970s, during which state health care costs skyrocketed. State governments began examining different ways to cut health care spending, and generic drugs seemed to be one viable solution. Meanwhile, pharmacists also softened their stance on generic drugs and substitutions, becoming more agreeable to their distribution. Kentucky became the first state to abolish its antisubstitution law, and by the mid-1980s, all fifty states legalized generic drug substitution. This came about, in part, due to the Drug Price Competition and Patent Term Restoration Act of 1984, better known as the Hatch-Waxman Act (H-W Act) after its Congressional sponsors (Gregory, 2016).

The H-W Act attempted to balance two issues in the pharmaceutical industry: the interests of the brand manufacturers and those of the generic producers (Gregory, 2016). The legislation was geared to encourage the brand-name manufacturers to continue investing in research and development of new drugs, while promoting generic drug competition in the marketplace, in an attempt to reduce the prices of drugs and to lower consumer costs. To do this, the act created a process by which drugs previously determined to be safe and effective could avoid the typically lengthy process of bringing a drug to market when it was to become a generic equivalent. Basically, it relaxed the testing requirements for generic manufacturers, meaning they could affordably enter the market in less time than what was required for the original brand-name drug.

These days, generics are routinely prescribed for various ailments and have been used, in many cases, as less-expensive alternative to the higher-cost brand-name pharmaceuticals. This doesn't mean all is well on the substitution front, however. Given the fragmented nature of many health care legislation issues, state policies, rules, and regulations pertaining to generics in lieu of brand names wildly differ. Attempts by federal legislators to enforce a minimum standard of generic drug substitution continue to be voted down, with politics of substitution continuing to play out at the state level. One state might be more lenient to distribution of generic drugs, while another could be somewhat more restrictive. It all depends.

Furthermore, physicians in all states can block generic substitutions by checking a box on their prescription forms that reads "dispense as written." If those physicians are being encouraged by brand-name manufacturers to *not* substitute generic drugs, that little box will likely remain unchecked. I already pointed out that physicians can be incentivized to direct patients to pricier alternatives.

Finally, even with concerns over higher drug prices, and media and legislative spotlights on the fact this is going on, the industry lobbyists and trade organizations continue to voice loud objections to generic substitutions. For instance, the AMA and Pharmaceutical Research and Manufacturers of America continue to oppose government intervention in the generic drug market, such as voting in and supporting stronger substitution laws and measures to prevent large price increases. This, in part, is preventing the market from truly determining whether generics could be a cost-saving method in the battle against higher drug prices.

◆ But Are They Really Less Expensive?

Then we come to the question as to how effective generic substitutions actually might be in controlling overall pharmaceutical costs for the consumer, even assuming the willingness of trade organizations and lobbyists to back off their antigeneric stance.

In theory, a generic should be able to sell for a fraction of the cost, for the following reasons:

- It is relatively inexpensive to bring a bioequivalent to market.
- The market for the drug typically already exists, meaning marketing expenses are considerably reduced.
- Because generics aren't restrained by patents, more manufacturers can come into the space, meaning more supply and downward pressure on pricing.

But let's examine these reasons and see if these theories actually hold up to reality.

Inexpensive to Bring to Market

In a free-market arena (i.e., a competitive market), when a price for a product is too high, another manufacturer could start to produce and offer a good at a lower price. But it has been pointed out, again and again, that there is no way in which the pharmaceutical industry operates in a capitalistic, free market, despite protests to the contrary. Furthermore, a generic manufacture just can't set up shop and begin cranking out pills once a patent expires on a drug. Generic drugmakers also have to undergo an approval process for bioequivalence drugs, meaning approval and sale of such pharmaceuticals is limited to the speed of the FDA review (Greene, Anderson, and Sharfstein, 2016). Before approval, that manufacturer needs to prove that the drug is safe and effective, which is required for any new drug that comes on the market. This, of course, takes time, which is compounded as the FDA is faced with continual backlogs when it comes to approving generic drug applications. Still, because generic manufacturers don't have to deal with development or research costs, it can be far less to bring such a drug to market versus its name-brand counterpart. The problem lies in getting the drugs approved and through the FDA backlog.

Reduced Marketing Expenses

When pharma companies first release drugs, promotional activities ramp up. Direct-to-consumer ads, along with aggressive practices in targeting health care providers, is on the top of the list as manufacturers work to recoup initial costs. As the product's lifecycle matures, advertising continues, mainly to keep reminding target markets that a drug is available to assist with everything from depression to rheumatoid arthritis and high cholesterol. Once the drug's patent expires and its market exclusivity has ended for a few years, it stands to reason that the market has matured and the drug will end up reduced in price, possibly due to competition or a generic equivalent making it to the market.

But as is consistently stressed throughout this paper, the pharmaceutical industry doesn't operate like that. Markets for some drugs can remain active long after a patent has expired. When examining drugs such as amoxicillin, we see at least ten different manufacturers for these pills. In order to recoup their manufacturing expenses, these generic manufacturers need to continue marketing their products. While the average consumer won't see television or magazine ads for these drugs, you'd better believe that pharmaceutical representatives are still paying visits to health care providers in hopes of encouraging the prescribing of these same-but-different drugs.

Furthermore, the marketing budgets of these companies might not be as large as those found through AstraZeneca, Pfizer, or Johnson & Johnson. As a result, the lack of "gloss" could make the drug "less cool" to patients and consumers. The "coolness" factor is important here and is the same with any product. People will naturally gravitate to the product that has all the air and ad time and carries the slicker packaging. Even in a side-by-side comparison of ingredients of a product, consumers simply trust the brand name more—because it is a brand name. This is just human nature.

But the not-so-fast acceptance of a generic drug means more effort needs to be directed to the middlemen—the insurance companies, PBMs, and prescribing health care providers—to ensure that patients are made aware of the idea that there is a generic brand available and that the generics are just as safe, if less costly, than the more expensive, brand-name drug.

◆ The Competitive Factor

Perhaps the main issue when it comes to generic drugs—and one reason why generics are being put forward as a viable option for reducing drug prices—is because of the law of supply and demand, as found through economics 101. Under this law, it would be assumed that the more generics that come on the market, the higher degree the competition. In reality, generic drugs have actually experienced a *decrease* in competition in recent years, due to factors such as supply-chain disruptions, FDA regulation loopholes, tough market conditions that drive companies out of business, mergers and acquisitions, and backlogs in processing generic drug applications by the FDA. In some extreme cases, reduced competition has led to individual companies actually being able to increase the prices of generic drugs. This was not at all what anyone had in mind when it came to use of generic drugs to control pharmaceutical pricing.

Let's take a look at the antibiotic doxycycline, which has been around for more than fifty years and is available through several manufacturers (Mui, 2019). This drug is commonly prescribed for a variety of bacterial infections and is generally the first-choice drug to treat everything from Lyme disease to urinary tract infections and even chlamydia. In 2011, the retail price of the generic version of this drug increased by 1,854 percent (Mui, 2019). Fast-forwarding a couple of years, the cost of five hundred doxycycline capsules increased from $20 in October 2013 to $1,028 by April 2014. Adding to this issue is that the price isn't all that consistent, based on the variation of doxycycline, how it is packaged, and where it is sold (Mui, 2019).

Another example involves common medications for cholesterol and high blood pressure. For example, the price on a one-year supply of the cholesterol-lowering drug pravastatin rose from $27 to $196 during the same period. Some might know this drug under the brand name of Pravachol.

There are a few reasons why competition might be so great when it comes to generic drugs. First, much as is the case for brand-name drugs, this is a high-barriers-to-entry industry, even when it comes to manufacturing generics. The manufacturing process for generics isn't all that different from brand-name manufacturing; it requires a huge capital investment in equipment, facilities, and staff to run it all. Because of this, even the older, more established generic medications might be produced by only one or two manufacturers (Greene, Anderson, and Sharfstein, 2016). They are the ones that already have the resources in place to do this.

Aside from leading to potential shortages of a particular drug, manufacturing problems at a single generic facility can really put a kink in the national supply of a drug. If this should happen, "gray-market distributors" can hop in and increase drug prices. Gray marketeers are not illegal, but they can do a number when it comes to drug pricing.

Gray markets involve the sale and trading of pharmaceuticals that have been stockpiled by wholesale distributors versus the original manufacturers (Hemphill, 2016). The distributors are the ones who set the prices, rather than the original manufacturers. Though legal, this activity is unofficial, unauthorized, and unintended by the original manufacturer.

Finally, drug shortages, especially in a time of need, can lead to price gouging.

Adding insult to the price issue is the danger to quality. Drugs bought and stockpiled by wholesalers (and even pharmacies) mean that, between manufacturer and consumer, that product could change hands up to five times, during which it might be repackaged and relabeled, stored under poor conditions, or even replaced by counterfeits (Hemphill, 2016).

Finally, it goes without saying that Big Pharma isn't all that thrilled with the idea of competition coming in to steal profits—or market share—away. These companies do what they can to hang on to their patents for as long as possible.

◆ The Evergreen Factor

"Evergreen" has a variety of definitions, depending on the industry that is being discussed. In the pharmaceutical industry, and in the case of brand-name and generic drug manufacturing, evergreening allows pharmaceutical companies to both extend their monopolies on drugs and to hold off generic competition by obtaining patents that cover new uses for drugs, as well as allowing for different manufacturing methods and formulations (DeArment, 2018). One of the better-known examples of this technique is pharmaceutical manufacturer Pfizer and its development and sale of Lyrica.

In 1995, Pfizer filed a patent on its neuropathic pain drug pregabalin, marketed under the brand name of Lyrica (I-MAK, 2018). The medication was approved by the FDA in 2007 to treat fibromyalgia syndrome (FMS), being the first drug approved to treat and manage this disease (Boomershine, 2010). FMS is a disease involving widespread pain, tender points on the body, fatigue, depression, anxiety, and nonrestorative sleep, among other symptoms.

Before being used to manage symptoms of FMS, pregabalin had been FDA approved for treating diabatic peripheral neuropathic pain and postherpetic neuralgia and was used as an adjunctive therapy among adult patients suffering from partial onset seizures.

Its use as a management drug for FMS came as a relief for those with the disease, who were unable to obtain relief from other methods. The drug has been a major source of revenue for Pfizer, grossing more than $5 billion in global sales in 2017, with $3 billion of that coming from US payers, including private insurance companies, Medicare, and Medicaid (I-MAK, 2018). Part of the commercial success of the product was driven by the 163 percent price increases over a six-year period, along with millions spent by Pfizer on direct-to-consumer advertising (I-MAK, 2018). There is nothing wrong with this. But the story becomes more interesting, the older Lyrica becomes.

Lyrica was scheduled to go off patent at the end of 2018, with the entry of generic competition potentially reducing Pfizer's revenue from the drug by up to 90 percent in less than two years (I-MAK, 2018). But Pfizer filed for, and won, a six-month pediatric exclusivity extension for Lyrica in late 2018, after testing the drug in patients with pediatric epilepsy (Saganowsky, 2018).

Pfizer was able to do this because of another federal blessing. Drug patents can get extensions of up to five years and then an additional six-month extension if the pharma manufacturer conducts studies on the drug's suitability for use in children (Engelberg, 2015). Pfizer, not being any fool, tested the drug in younger patients, providing the impetus to file for additional patent protection.

The company filed, and was issued, patents for an additional twenty-year period on a controlled-release formulation of the product dubbed Lyrica CR (I-MAK, 2018). The new product meant patients could take a single pill per day versus the two or three they took under the older drug (I-MAK, 2018). "With these patents, Pfizer's hold on the market will remain and, if history is a guide, they will continue major repeated increases in the price of the drug," according to the nonprofit group Medicines, Access, and Knowledge (I-MAK).

Interestingly enough, things were different in the United Kingdom, in which Pfizer lost its patent fight with that country's Supreme Court (Saganowsky, 2018). The high court ruled that Lyrica's neuropathic pain patent claims were invalid, following a dispute of several years, allowing NHS Engliahs to potentially re-coup £502 million in overspending (Saganowsky, 2018).

And patients who don't mind taking two or three pregabalin tablets a day will have some generic options. When the initial patent "officially" ran out in June 2019, the FDA approved generic versions, with nine pharmaceutical companies authorized to begin manufac-turing and marketing the drug (Chase, 2019). There are also viable, approved generic and brand alternatives to treat FMS, including gabapentin, duloxetine, savella, and amitriptyline, the latter of which is an older antidepressant that is sometimes used for nerve pain (Chase, 2019). As such, there are alternatives that patients can rely on, assuming, of course, that they know to ask (and that their phy-sicians agree).

However, Pfizer's evergreening its Lyrica means that doctors can still prescribe the extended-release brand-name version, and if patients don't know any better (or don't do their research), they'll go along with it. Nor is Pfizer the only one involved with the evergreen process.

Evergreening means new uses could require FDA approvals, as is what happened when Pfizer asked for the Lyrica patent extension to treat childhood epilepsy (DeArment, 2018). Even something as min-ute as small-molecule changes could lead to a new patent. Changing the shape of a pill, its color, or even its size could mean a new patent and more years of continued monopoly on a drug. And all of this is perfectly OK. It also blocks the potential generic—and less expensive—drug from coming on to the market.

This leads to another tool used by Big Pharma, known as "product hopping." This happens when a company introduces minor changes to a branded drug, before the expiration on its monopoly protection (Khullar and Bach, 2020). To do this, the company physically removes the original product from the market while making the changes. The result is that generic drug approvals and substitutions are additionally delayed (Khullar and Bach, 2020). The FDA could put an end to this by not granting market exclusivity to a drug's cosmetic differences. Meanwhile, the Federal Trade Commission could (and has not done so yet) step in to more aggressively enforce antitrust laws against such tactics (Khullar and Bach, 2020).

Furthermore, the manufacturing process for biologics, versus pharmaceuticals, don't have an expiration date on patents. Again, biologics are manufactured from "live" cells, or organisms, meaning their production is less easy to copy. Along these lines, the manufacturing processes for biologics are trade secrets, meaning even an enterprising generic pharmaceutical manufacturer wouldn't be able to do an apples-to-apples creation of the product.

I-MAK, in a 2018 report, pointed out that the top-grossing drugs have, on average, 125 patent applications filed to extend their commercial monopolies beyond the average twenty years of protection. The report went on to suggest that the filings allow pharmaceutical manufacturers to increase the price of their branded drugs by an average of 68 percent over a six-year period while stalling generic competition by an average of thirty-eight years (I-MAK, 2018). The following chart lists the twelve drugs I-MAK studied and the patents filed to extend the pharmaceutical manufacturers' hold on the market:

Company/ Drug	Condition Treated	Number of Patent Applications	Number of Patents Issued	Price Change Since 2012	Years Blocking Competition	On the US Market Since
AbbVie/ Humira	Arthritis	247	132	+144%	29	2002
Biogen-Genetech/ Rituxan	Cancer	204	94	+25%	47	1997
Celgene/ Revlimid	Multiple Myeloma	106	96	+79%	40	2005
Amgen/Enbrel	Arthritis	57	41	+155%	39	1998
Roche-Genetech/ Herceptin	Cancer	186	108	-58%	48	1998
Pfizer-BMS/ Eliquis	Stroke/ Embolism	48	27	+69%	34	2012
Johnson & Johnson/ Remicade	Arthritis	123	66	+18%	32	1998
Roche/Avastin	Cancer	219	86	+16%	43	2004
Johnson & Johnson/ Xarelto	Blood Clogs	49	30	+87%	31	2011
Bayer-Regeneron/ Eylea	Macular Degeneration	67	51	+6%	34	2018
Sanofi/Lantus	Diabetes	74	49	+114%	37	2000
Pfizer/Lyrica	Pain	118	68	+163%	32	2004

(I-MAK, 2018)

At least pregabalin has some competition, and some manufacturers have started manufacturing generics against Lyrica. But getting back to the issue of Daraprim, with which this paper was started, the drug itself (pyrimethamine) had been eligible for generic development for close to half a century. However, no generic drug had entered the market from the time when it was first released to the time in which Turing Pharmaceuticals/Vyera Pharmaceuticals increased the price (Marciarille, 2017). There is no specific reason why a generic hadn't been released up to that point, other than the ones already mentioned: manufacturer loopholes, an incredibly long FDA process, and a process that impeded generic manufacturers from actually getting samples of the brand medication needed to develop a generic.

This particular action—and example—demonstrates that the cost of a modestly valued drug may be substantially enhanced by a drug distribution mechanism that defeats generic entry. It's highly that a generic entry, or any other competition, for that matter, could lower the price of a drug such as Daraprim, so long as the new entry is "timely, likely and sufficient." In the case of Daraprim, however, is that a competing generic entry would not have been considered timely, from the point of view of drug costs, due to the price spike of the drug itself. Only time will tell if a generic can substantially lower the price of pyrimethamine. In February 2020, the FDA finally approved the first generic of Daraprim for treatment of toxoplasmosis (FDA (b), 2020).

◆ Reverse Payments

The Sherman Antitrust Act, as it pertains to the pharmaceutical industry, specifically prohibits agreements among competitors that "unreasonably restrain trade" as such agreements tend to benefit the producers rather than consumers or market forces. There are two types of "unreasonable" agreements: agreements between parties on the same level of production (horizontal agreements) and agreements taking place between parties at different levels of the supply chain (vertical agreements).

Manufacturers in the pharmaceutical industry will sometimes embark on what are known as "reverse payments," otherwise known as "pay-for-delay" agreements, which can appear in a settlement of a patent litigation between a brand-name manufacturer and generic drug producer (Gregory, 2016; Kantarjian, Steensma, Sanjuan, Elshaug, and Light, 2014). This, in a sense, is when generic manufacturers figuratively get into bed with the brand-name pharma manufacturer.

Such patent litigation can, in fact, be common. In many cases, brand and generic manufacturers can enter closed-door settlement agreements or negotiations, which divide the market for a particular drug (Gregory, 2016). This happens when a generic manufacturer submits a Paragraph IV certification with the FDA before a patent expires, giving the brand-name manufacturer forty-five days to file a patent infringement lawsuit (Gregory, 2016). Under a reverse-payment agreement, the generic receives a benefit (i.e., payment) from the brand holder for its agreement not to enter the market. Such agreements are considered a "win-win" for both brand-name manufacturers and their generic counterparts (FTC, 2010). Pharmaceutical prices remain high, while both the brand-name and generic manufacturers share the benefits of monopolized profits (FTC, 2010).

Certainly, the FTC has condemned reverse-payment schemes as illegal under antitrust doctrines. The problem, however, is that in the case *FTC v. Actavis,* the US Supreme Court failed to define the term "settlement." While the court indicated that "cash reverse-payment settlements between patent holders and generic manufacturers violate antitrust laws," the ruling of the case said nothing about non-monetary value settlements (Gregory, 2016). An example of such a settlement is an unauthorized generic agreement in which the brand holder agrees not to bring its own authorized generic to the market so that the generic "partner" can have exclusivity on its own delayed entry into the market.

Sadly, this type of agreement comes from a loophole in the H-W Act, which was created with the good intentions of bringing down the costs of drugs while working to not stifle innovation of drug brand holders.

◆ Different Generics

It's hard to believe, but there are even different kinds of generics when it comes to drugs. All generic drugs require approval by the FDA before they can be released for use to the market. The concept of "approved generic" drugs, sometimes known as "authorized generics," is a little different, however. An approved generic is an actual brand-name drug that is marketed and distributed without the actual brand name on the label (FDA (c), 2020). Such an approved generic might be marketed by either the brand-name drug company or by another company, with the brand company's permission—and it's all perfectly legal. This adds more confusion to an already very confusing process.

◆ Generics Control Prices—Kind Of

From the point of view of the Federal Trade Commission, when it comes to generic drugs, the higher the number of generic entries, the better the overall price competition (Marciarille, 2017). This is especially the case if one follows the theories provided by supply and demand.

But once again, it's different when it comes to the pharmaceutical industry. When it comes to pharmaceutical generics, a sole-source price spike (such as that experienced by Daraprim), combined with a distribution mechanism in place that deliberately delays generic entries, means the FTC theory toward competition and antimonopolistic practices has definite flaws. Marciarille pointed out, for instance, that Turing's/Vyera's innovation wasn't so much involved with production and/or distribution of Daraprim as much as it involved "learning how to game the generic entrant system to delay or divert new entrants for an expensive interval" (p. 47). In other words, for generics to work as a price suppressant for pharmaceuticals, issues such as timely entry need to be addressed. Also needing to be addressed is a distribution system that is in place, by the industry, which deliberately suppresses any kind of competition.

There is, however, another aspect when it comes to generic pharmaceuticals and their pricing. Though it seems as though generic drugs have undergone price spikes in recent years, research shows that, in actuality, the chained, direct, out-of-pocket consumer price index for generics actually decreased by 50 percent between 2007 and 2016 (Frank, Hicks, and Berndt, 2019). Additionally, during the same time period, the total CPI for generic prescription drugs fell by nearly 80 percent.

This would be good news, except it isn't. Franks et al. (2019) indicate that while generic prescriptions are driving overall prices downward, those price declines aren't always passed through to consumers. "Our evidence suggests that overall affordability is not the main problem in the generic drug market," comment Frank and his fellow authors. And the reason for this is, once again, insurance companies and PBMs have been offering products that are increasingly shifting costs from insurers to consumers. As a result, consumers are experiencing a greater share of generic drug costs, even as the overall price for generic drugs has dropped and continues to drop. This led the researchers to suggest "a closer look at the workers of the entire generic drug supply chain (manufacturer, wholesaler, pharmaceutical benefit manager, insurance, and retailer)."

As such, the answer as to whether generic substitutions can actually reduce prices is somewhat of a mixed bag. Because the pharmaceutical industry operates in a highly monopolistic environment, one in which patents and other issues can delay the entry of competition, it's difficult to say if no-name brands, overall, can reduce costs. Furthermore, the degree to which savings can be realized isn't in the hands of the manufacturers but is dependent on private insurance plans and PBMs. Again, generics are just one solution, but because of industry complexity, it isn't working as well as it could. Still, if there is any good news, it's that many consumers are realizing some cost savings by going off brand.

HIGHER DRUG PRICES AND THEIR IMPACTS

UP UNTIL NOW, WE'VE FOCUSED ON HOW BIG PHARMA IS benefitting from the current legal and so-called "competitive" structure when it comes to manufacturing, distributing, and profiting from drugs. We also took a deep dive into the massive complexity that makes up this industry and the stakeholders involved. What we haven't examined so far, however, is the impact of these practices on a rather important stakeholder: the consumer.

As such, it's a good idea to take a look at how Big Pharma's—and others'—practices are affecting those end users. These are the consumers who rely on these drugs to alleviate painful and debilitating conditions and, in many cases, to stay alive. While senior citizens and lower-income families tend to be the ones who suffer most from these higher prices and monopolistic practices evidenced by the industry, higher drug prices have a dire impact on US society, as a whole. In this section, I delve more deeply into just how escalating pharmaceutical prices are having a negative effect on members of our society. If such an effect continues, it could spell additional costs and more problems for the future.

◆ Senior Citizens

As mentioned earlier in this paper, life spans have increased. At the turn of the twentieth century, one in forty Americans died on an annual basis (Penn Wharton, 2016). By 2013, that rate fell to one in 140 Americans, a cumulative improvement of more than two-thirds. Additionally, life expectancy at birth increased by more than thirty years over the same time period, from forty-seven years old to seventy-nine years old. The reason why we started viewing longer expectancies was due to public health measures and better nutrition, which helped lead to reductions in mortality, especially when it came to infectious diseases.

Over the past fifty-five years, between 1960 and 2015, overall life expectancy in the United States increased by almost a decade, from 69.7 years (1960) to 79.4 years (Medina, Sabo, and Vespa, 2020). The largest gains in life expectancy took place between 1970 and 1980, a fact attributable to increases in vaccines, decreases in infectious diseases and cardiovascular problems and mortalities, and prevention programs related to smoking, alcohol consumption, and promotion of physical activity. As such, mortality improvements since the mid-twentieth century have been driven mainly by better disease management and treatment (Penn Wharton, 2016). By "treatment" we mean lifestyle changes and medication management. By 2060, life expectancy for the total US population is projected to increase by about six years, from 79.7 in 2017 to 85.6 (Medina, Sabo, and Vespa, 2020). The upshot of this is Americans are living to greater ages, and this trend is likely to continue.

There is a dual-edge sword to this news, however. Americans are living longer, thanks to better disease management, courtesy of state-of-the-art medical technology and specialty drugs. The cardiovascular event or cancer diagnosis likely to carry off great-grandfather in 1905 can now be controlled by beta blockers, at-home chemotherapy treatments, calcium channel blockers, ACE inhibitors, and diuretics. But this disease management—and overall survival—comes at a cost. Older Americans dependent on pharmaceuticals and specialty drugs are finding themselves in the crosshairs of higher health care and drug prices. This can especially be a problem for senior citizens on fixed incomes who suddenly find themselves unable to afford medications on which they depend to survive or to have some semblance of a decent quality of life.

KFF's 2019 Health Tracking Poll indicated that nearly nine out of ten adults age sixty-five and older reported they are taking prescription medication (Kirzinger, Neuman, Cubanski, and Brodie, 2019). This breaks down to the following:

- three-fourths of 50-64-year-olds surveyed are taking prescription drugs
- half of 30-49-year-olds are taking those medications
- four in ten 18-29-year-olds are taking prescription drugs

Additionally, older adults are more likely than their younger counterparts to be taking multiple prescription medications (Kirzinger, Neuman, Cubanski, and Brodie, 2019). And the majority of those who are older than age sixty-five are getting some form of help from Medicare Part D. But this was not always the case.

The Struggles of Prescription Drug Legislation

Anyone looking at the history of health care legislation—of any kind—is likely struck by the huge difficulty it is to get any kind of legislation passed to protect people. This has been the case when it comes to nationalized health care. Even the most recent act passed, the Patient Protection and Affordable Care Act of 2010, keeps ending up challenged in court. Passing that legislation also required a year-long effort focused on town halls, negotiations, and campaigns against misinformation and wrong news (such as "granny panels" and rationed health care). For some odd reason, anytime anyone mentions legislating health care, cries of "socialism" abound, which effectively shuts down many efforts.

One such effort that did make it through—only barely, and with a whole lot of horse-trading on President Lyndon Johnson's part—was the Medicare Act. This was enacted in 1965 as part of the Title XVIII of the Social Security Act and was originally envisioned with two parts. Part A focused on hospital coverage, while part B took care of supplementary medical insurance. This latter would have also included an outpatient prescription drug benefit (Oliver, Lee, and Lipton, 2004). The prescription benefit, however, was dropped from Part B as it was considered too unpredictable and carrying too high a price tag. Ironically enough, the Medicaid program, enacted as Title XIX of the Social Security Act (which I will discuss in more detail below), provided more comprehensive drug coverage for the indigent elderly, along with those who are blind and disabled, as well as eligible, lower-income families with dependent children. The Medicaid program included outpatient prescription drug coverage as an optional benefit. All states elected to offer it when they set up Medicaid programs.

This is not to suggest that Medicare covered no prescription drugs. It did, as long as those drugs were dispensed in doctors' offices rather than self-administered by patients. This provision had been enacted less out of concern about patients paying higher drug costs and more out of practicality. Doctors had been putting patients into hospitals to ensure they would receive the medications they needed, as the prescriptions were covered for hospital patients. It was believed that allowing doctors to administer the drugs to patients, in their offices, would lower overall drug costs. Over the years, as physicians' offices were added to the list under Medicare, with members of Congress continuing to add amendments allowing Medicare coverage for specific drugs manufactured by pharmaceutical companies in their districts. By 2001, Medicare had covered approximately 454 physician-dispensed prescription drugs, at a cost of $6.5 billion a year, an increase from the $700 million reported in 1992. The problem, however, was obvious. Patients would need to make unnecessary trips to their providers' offices, just to obtain coverage for specific drugs.

From Medicare enactment in 1965 to passage of the Medicare Prescription Drug, Improvement and Modernization Act (MMA) of 2003, policy makers tried several times to introduce prescription drug coverage under Medicare, only to be thwarted by lobbyists and, in one case, the economy. President Jimmy Carter had thought to address the topic of Medicare prescription coverage during the 1970s. However, a poor economy, rife with inflation, stagflation, and continued runaway gas prices, put his priorities in other areas, and the Medicare issue was shelved for several years.

The Medicare Catastrophic Coverage Act of 1988 saw passage of increased prescription coverage in which Medicare would cover 80 percent of drug costs, once the patient met the $600 deductible (Oliver, Lee, and Lipton, 2004). The problem, however, was that financing the plan meant an increase in the Part B premium as well as a "supplemental premium" on the amount of federal income taxes owed, above $150. This, and other issues, led to calls to repeal MCCA, especially after the Congressional Budget Office released projections showing that the costs of the act—and beneficiaries' costs for the self-financing program—were expected to be far higher than initial projections. Congress ended up repealing most of the MCCA's major provisions in 1989, including the prescription drug benefit.

The following decade, Medicare prescription drug benefits were dealt another blow when President Bill Clinton's major proposals for health care reform died in the mid-1990s (Oliver, Lee, and Lipton, 2004). While the defeat of the reform wasn't related to prescription drug coverage, the provisions provoked concerns among pharmaceutical firms that drug benefits might be accompanied by price controls and other regulations. Later in the decade, the growing availability of Medicare-managed care plans, combined with projected budget surpluses (due to the Balanced Budget Act of 1997), led to questions about why the government couldn't help cover prescription drug costs for Medicare beneficiaries. The political pressure to expand coverage continued as many private insurance companies withdrew from the Medicare+Choice program in 1999, meaning millions were forced to shop elsewhere for prescription drug benefits; many of these benefits were not affordable.

It wasn't until early 2003—when Republicans had control of the House, Senate, and presidency, that a focus on prescription coverage for Medicare beneficiaries came about. The final product—the 678-page Medicare Prescription Drug, Improvement and Modernization Act—passed in 2003, after a great deal of political wrangling. The two main, better-known points of the bill were as follows:

- Most beneficiaries had to choose between existing drug coverage or joining a new Medicare Part D program through stand-alone drug plans or through comprehensive plans under Part C (which was renamed the Medicare Advantage Program).
- Part D beneficiaries would pay an initial premium of $35 per month and a $250 annual deductible. Medicare would pay 75 percent of annual expenses between $250 and $2,250 for approved prescription drugs, nothing for expenses between $2,250 and $5,100, and 95 percent of expenses above $5,100. Known as the "doughnut hole," it meant beneficiaries were responsible for $420 in premiums, $1,590 out of pocket to reach the initial breakeven point, and $4,020 of the first $5,100 in annual drug expenses.

The goal was to directly benefit low-income Medicare beneficiaries with no supplemental source of insurance coverage through retiree benefits, Medigap plans, or Medicaid. Even getting this bill approved took a great deal of time and political muscle—and even with all of that, it barely squeaked through, with Congress voting to approve down political lines.

Perhaps unsurprisingly, the pharmaceutical industry loved the new act in that there was no direct administration of benefits by the federal government, no explicit cost control measures, and no legalization of drug reimportation (Oliver, Lee, and Lipton, 2004). Furthermore, the bill did nothing to control the out-of-control prices of drugs. As such, the companies breathed a sigh of relief and continued to set their own prices on drugs.

Older People Still Pay a Lot

Here's the problem. Even with involvement of Medicare Part D, drugs are still hugely expensive because the act didn't address the problem it needed to, namely the cause of higher prices as opposed to what could be covered. Research presented by AARP reported that brand-name drug prices increased more than twice as fast as inflation on a year-over-year basis; retail prices for 267 widely used brand-name prescription drugs increased by 5.8 percent, versus the general inflation of 2.4 percent over the same period (in 2018) (Schondelmeyer and Purvis, 2019). Interestingly enough, the report also noted that, while twice as high as inflation, the increase was the slowest average annual price increase for widely used brand-name prescription drugs in more than a decade. The good news is, therefore, that prices are still going up, but not as quickly as they did. Still, for more than a decade, annual brand-name drug price increases exceeded the general inflation rate by from twofold to more than a hundredfold, with the average cost for one brand-name medication used on a chronic basis being more than $7,200. This metric, re-ported for 2018, was almost four times higher than in 2006. While Medicare coverage is supposed to help lower drug prices for ben-eficiaries, that lack of a price control isn't doing a very good job of keeping such costs in line.

While various legislation since the narrow passage of the Medicare Modernization Act has managed to shrink the infamous "doughnut hole," Part D has no cap on out-of-pocket drug costs (unlike what is offered through private insurance plans) (Andrews, 2019). In 2019, Medicare beneficiaries pay 25 percent of the price of their brand-name drugs, until they reach $5,100 in out-of-pocket costs. Once that amount is reached, the catastrophic portion kicks in and the cost drops to 5 percent, but it never goes away. While 5 percent might not seem a lot, for some drugs—such as Copaxone—which cost about $75,000 annually, this can be a great deal. Capaxone is used to treat some forms of multiple sclerosis and can reduce the frequency of re-lapses. But the structure of Medicare, combined with the high price for this drug, meant that one MS patient, who wanted to retire but can't, paid $2,700 before catastrophic coverage kicked in plus an additional $2,950 owed for the remainder of the year. "I feel like I'm being punished financially for having a chronic disease," said the patient, who is sixty-six years old (Andrews, 2019). He is also con-sidering discontinuing Capaxone to save money. Discontinuing this medication could lead to more relapses and eventual hospitalization, probably sooner than this patient would have wanted or was needed.

The same holds true for cancer patients taking chemotherapy pills. Once upon a time, chemotherapy was administered in hospitals or clinics; many forms of chemo still are administered in this way.

But the new drugs on the market allow patients to receive chemo without the bother of going to a clinic or hospital. The problem, however, is that this "convenience" comes with a price, especially among Medicare recipients on a fixed income. One such patient, who took Ibrance to keep her breast cancer in check, paid $2,200 for two months, with the cost dropping to $584 per month for treatment. Ironically enough, if she were getting traditional drug infusions in a hospital or clinic instead of taking the oral medication, Medicare Part B would kick in and co-insurance payments would be covered.

Much like the patient with MS is considering other senior citizens just go without the drug, a 2018 survey, spearheaded by UpWell Health, reported that 45 percent of respondents with diabetes went without care at some point, due to the cost of insulin (Caffrey, 2018). Again, there is no generic equivalent for insulin but plenty of brand-name (and seemingly expensive) versions. Additionally, during that same year, the American Diabetes Association reported that the annual average costs for diabetes care was $7,900 per year.

The above stories support the 2019 KHN poll, indicating that while a majority of older adults have prescription coverage through Medicare Part D, most older adults believe the cost of prescription drugs is unreasonable. The poll also uncovered the following results (Kirzinger, Neuman, Cubanski, and Brodie, 2019):

- One-fourth of older adults who take prescription drugs say it is difficult to afford these drugs, with one in ten saying that it is "very difficult."
- Those who report being either in "only fair" or "poor" health, whose household income is less than $30,000 annually, and

who take four or more prescription drugs are more likely to report difficulties in affording the drugs.

- Approximately one in five older adults report not talking medicines as prescribed at some point in the previous year, due to the cost. This includes those reporting that they haven't filled a prescription, took an over-the-counter drug instead, cut pills in half, or skipped a dose.

- Among those who report not taking their medications as prescribed, slightly more than half said they didn't tell their health care provider. In addition, one-fifth of this group said their conditions got worse as a result of not taking their prescription as recommended.

- While seven in ten older adults say they will talk to their doctors or health care providers about safety of drugs and their potential side effects (for a new medication), approximately four in ten older adults say they usually talk to their doctors about whether there is a less-expensive alternative. Furthermore, just over one-third discuss the cost they would have to pay for a new medication.

- The majority of older adults support various actions aimed at keeping costs down, including international reference pricing, proposals to allow the federal government to negotiate price spending, and bipartisan proposals to add a cap on out-of-pocket spending.

In focusing on older Americans, the AARP's research, mentioned before, pointed out that for older Americans, who take an average of 4.5 brand-name prescription drugs on a chronic basis, the average annual cost of therapy would have been more than $32,000 in 2018, almost 25 percent higher than the median annual income for Medicare beneficiaries, which was $26,200 (Schondelmeyer and Purvis, 2019).

The report went on to suggest that such spending increases and growing drug prices would affect all Americans ultimately. "Those with private health coverage will pay more in cost-sharing and higher premiums for their health coverage," the report pointed out. "In addition, increased government spending will ultimately lead to higher taxes and/or cuts to public programs." It goes without saying that the higher the drug prices go, the more health insurance companies, run through Medicare, are putting on the consumer. Such cost-sharing, incidentally, is a hallmark of the US health care system. Other industrialized nations don't require this type of arrangement.

Adding insult to this pot of high-price injury is that older citizens are consistently exposed to ongoing pharmaceutical advertising, especially on TV (Alpert, Lakdawalla, and Snood, 2015). One estimate points out that adults aged fifty and above (which also happens to be a population with a high rate of prescription drug use) watch an average of more than forty hours of live television a week. This target audience, in a sense, is a sitting duck when it comes to slick promotions and promises of better health. This in turn means that pharmaceutical advertising can have a persuasive impact on specific drug use/drug prescriptions.

Researchers have determined that drug utilization tends to be highly responsive to advertising; following Part D implementation, there was a 6 percent increase in the average number of prescriptions purchased by the nonelderly in areas with high elderly share, relative to areas that had low elderly share. Basically, advertising increases take-up of drug treatments; on the positive side, it does improve compliance for existing patients. It also can help older people become more aware of potential treatments and outcomes that might be helpful for chronic issues, such as arthritis.

The problem, however, is that among those elderly who might not have as much money, advertising adds to costs of brand-name medications which can, in turn, mean unaffordable drugs for the elderly US population. And if the elderly population can't afford the drugs it sees advertised on television, it is likely to go without. This can create even more problems down the road.

Drug Discontinuance and Nonadherence

The problem when senior citizens—or anyone else, for that matter—don't take their prescribed medicines, a practice known as nonadherence, is that it doesn't save the health care system much in the way of money. Certainly, someone who doesn't take his or her pills can save a little bit of money, especially if that individual is living on a tight budget. But from a big-picture perspective, non-adherence ends up leading to worse problems down the road in the form of increased complications and hospitalizations (Rosenbaum and Shrank, 2013). When people can't afford the cost of taking the medications prescribed for them, visits to emergency departments increase as do hospitalizations (Brody, 2017). Even without hospitalization or ER visits, nonadherence affects quality of life. People with rheumatoid arthritis don't end up in the emergency room unless they are in horrible pain. But not having the right medicine, due to high costs, can make these individuals very uncomfortable and not able to function.

It's been found that medication adherence tends to drop when the copay for a drug is $50 or higher; this is the same with the higher-priced biologics. Unfortunately, cutting medical dosages in half or skipping doses altogether reduces the effectiveness of drugs, meaning higher medical bills if, and when, a health emergency occurs. And again, it increases discomfort in a population that is already experiencing the aches and pains of old age.

This isn't necessarily an individual problem, as much as it is a public health and societal problem. Specifically, nonadherence costs the United States an estimated $100 billion to $290 billion annually (Rosenbaum and Shrank, 2013). This makes sense. The cost of an emergency room visit from someone who can't really afford it has to be paid by someone. That "someone" is generally people who have higher-cost premiums. As such, the issue is both that of patient affordability as well as a system-wide one. This is becoming more of an issue as Americans are getting older. Baby boomers, a high-count population, are entering their geriatric years, meaning high prices and nonadherence could likely continue to be a concern.

So to summarize, the issue of prescription drugs affecting senior citizens is that such drugs—especially specialty drugs—are keeping older people alive for longer. That's the good news. The bad news, however, is that various forms of legislation have been enacted to help boost prescription coverage for older people. But because of the politics of prescriptions, the legislation isn't doing a very good job of keeping the prices down. Namely because the legislation doesn't focus on price controls (out of fear of angering Big Pharma and lucrative political contributions). Nor does it put caps on spending. Instead, it just focuses on what is covered and what isn't, which does nothing to solve the overall problems of higher drug prices. This means that, for many older people, staying alive—or even having any kind of decent quality of life—is becoming a very expensive proposition.

◆ Lower-Income Families

It should come as no surprise that lower-income families also tend to be affected by higher prescription costs, especially when it comes to out-of-pocket issues. However, unlike Medicare, Medicaid's prescription drug benefit seems to be more effective. Similar to Medicare, Medicaid drug coverage relies on a complex formula of rebates and discounts, mired in the usual red tape. And once again, Medicaid legislation does nothing to control the problem of higher costs—in other words, no targeting of pharmaceutical company pricing practices or rebates to pharmacy benefit managers.

On the positive side, all states offer some kind of Medicaid coverage; Medicaid beneficiaries who also have Medicare receive their drug coverage through Medicare (KFF, 2019). While Medicaid drug spending growth has declined since 2014, policy makers are concerned about increased drug spending in the future. Due to the program's role in financing coverage for high-need populations, Medicaid pays a disproportionate share of certain high-cost specialty drugs (KFF, 2019). This includes the so-called "blockbuster" drugs (KFF, 2019).

The total amount paid by Medicaid for a particular drug is based on the following (KFF, 2019):

- Dispensing fees paid to pharmacists. Medicaid doesn't purchase drugs directly from manufacturers or wholesalers. The program pays for the cost of drugs dispensed to beneficiaries through pharmacies. Reimbursements are made based on the actual acquisition cost—or AAC—for a drug.

- Amount paid to the pharmacy for drug ingredients. Pharmacies that dispense drugs to Medicaid beneficiaries buy those drugs and ingredients from manufacturers, negotiating their prices. This is a proprietary process, with negotiations based on manufacturer-set list prices for a drug. The problem here, however, is that manufacturers don't provide public information about how they set list prices and haven't been required to explain changes in a product's list price. These affect Medicaid reimbursement schedules, as they are plugged into the AAC.

- Manufacturer rebates. Finally, federal law requires manufacturers who want drugs covered under Medicaid to rebate a portion of the drug payments to the government. In return, Medicaid is required to cover almost all FDA-approved drugs produced by those manufacturers. The rebate factors vary by type of drug, whether it is a brand-name or generic pharmaceutical. These rebates apply, whether a state pays for prescription drugs on a fee-for-service program or includes them in managed care plan capitation payments.

While states oversee the dispensing fees, federal requirements control the other two inputs. More good news here: most state Medicaid programs require a generic substitution, unless the prescriber insists that the brand-name drug is medically necessary (KFF, 2019). As a result, generic drugs have accounted for the vast majority of prescription drug volume in Medicaid from 2014 through 2017.

However, while generic pharmaceuticals account for much of the drug utilization under Medicaid plans, brand-name drugs account for most of the drug spending (KFF, 2019). According to KFF, this growth in brand spending is caused by the launch of expensive new drugs, as well as price increases for some brand-name drugs. Under this latter category is insulin; there are no genetic versions of insulin.

I am focusing on Medicaid in this section, as the program covers approximately one in five Americans, accounting for one-sixth of US health care spending (Ohn and Kaltenboeck, 2019). This means the program covers 21 percent of the overall population, serving those who are low income and who are unable to work due to a disability or medical condition (Ohn and Kaltenboeck, 2019). The best way to analyze prescription costs on lower-income populations is to take a look at Medicaid statistics, especially because Medicaid programs are required to balance their annual budgets, and they rely heavily on the Medicaid Drug Rebate Program (MDRP) mentioned above. While the MDRP requires programs to maintain an open formulary covering all of a manufacturer's drugs, recent attempts by states to close those formularies is suggesting that there is a lack of negotiating power, exposing Medicaid to higher prescription prices. The design of the MDRP means Medicaid programs are exposed to pricing decisions by other stakeholders, specifically other payers, pharmacy benefit managers, and pharmaceutical manufacturers. Under closed formularies, it's possible that Medicaid beneficiaries could suffer from restrictions to drugs they might need.

Furthermore, given the fragmented nature of Medicaid—it is a state-run program and requirements vary from state to state— it's difficult to make a blanket statement about Medicaid and drug. There are, however, some conclusions we can come to, based on a few studies.

Some years ago, a study focused on a new measure of medication affordability, one that examined out-of-pocket drug expenses, relative to available household resources (Briesacher et al., 2009). The study's authors pointed out, quite rightfully, that accessing certain prescription drugs and their treatments "may sometimes consume catastrophic proportions of available income" (Briesacher et al., 2009, p. 600). Studies have demonstrated that lower-income American households have been forced to either cut back on basic necessities (such as food) or take fewer medications than prescribed, due to out-of-pocket drug costs. Research has shown that even incomes at even 200 percent of the federal poverty level are hard-pressed to be stretched to meet basic living needs, let alone to cover increasing medication costs. The study in question pointed out that medication costs consumed the largest proportion of health care expenses, both for lower-income households without Medicaid and those with Medicaid.

The results of the 2000s study were introduced a few years later in a KFF issue brief indicating that low-income families and individuals ineligible for Medicaid will find affordable health coverage options limited (Majerol, Tobert, and Damico, 2016). Though some low-income workers might be offered coverage by employers, and those in states that have not expanded Medicaid might have access to premium subsidies within the health care marketplaces, such private insurance options often require premiums as well as cost-sharing in the form of deductibles, copayments, and co-insurance (Majerol, Tobert, and Damico, 2016).

But lower-income households have limited resources, to which they must allocate to competing necessities, such as housing, food, and transportation. Basically, food and shelter absolutely need to come first with this population; once those needs are met, there is clothing and maybe, if there is enough money, prescriptions drugs. Added to this is that average spending among these households tends to greatly exceed the average income, meaning they could accrue debt, even as they are earning their paychecks. And low-income households with Medicaid tend to spend a smaller portion of their annual budget on health care compared to non-Medicaid households. It's difficult to determine how much prescription drugs make up as part of this statistic. But it makes sense that if out-of-pocket prescription costs become costly, it's not difficult to imagine that a household might decide to do without the prescription, so as to put food on the table.

Then there is the other low-income cohort, namely those who earn too much to qualify for Medicaid but who don't have employer-covered health insurance or who can't afford their own. This could fit the profile of many part-time, hourly workers who are earning just enough to skirt over the Medicaid threshold but also can't afford the high potential costs of needed prescriptions. This population cohort is probably the most vulnerable as there are no safety nets available if they should need a drug but can't afford it (unless a clinic can provide the drug or a physician has free samples). Again, when families survive on tight budgets, an unexpected health cost—such a prescription—can put that budget in jeopardy. Nonadherence is more likely, which can hurt a person's health and quality of life. This adds insult to injury, as a lower-income person is already struggling in many areas.

And as mentioned above, nonadherence costs not just families but societies. The person who contracts pneumonia but can't afford to stay home and rest or get an antibiotic for treatment will become worse. This could lead to a hospitalization, which in turn puts more strain on the nation's health care system, not to mention the hospital's budget. An individual who can't afford a bottle of pills will certainly be unable to afford a hospital stay—meaning the hospital has to carry that charge on its books. The costs have to be made up somewhere, and they are; those who have private insurance are charged higher prices, simply because they can be. This in turn boosts health insurance premiums, making the cost of health care even higher.

Members of lower-income families battling wide ranges of cancers are especially at risk from high costs of pharmaceuticals. For instance, in 2012, twelve of the thirteen new drugs approved for cancer treatments were priced well above $100,000 per year of therapy (Kantarjian, Steensma, Sanjuan, Elshaug, and Light, 2014). Typical out-of-pocket expenses for such treatment end up being between $20,000 to $30,000 per year, which is close to half the average annual household income in the United States. This could also be the *entire* income of a lower-income family. Because of the costs, up to 20 percent of patients diagnosed with some form of cancer might either decide to not take the cancer treatments or could "compromise significantly on the treatment plan" (Kantarjian, Steensma, Sanjuan, Elshaug, and Light, 2014, p. e208). In other words, the potential for nonadherence, leading to difficulties down the road. And if those cancer patients are too wealthy for Medicaid but live on a very tight low-income budget, nonadherence becomes that much more likely. This creates additional medical problems—and a higher expense problem—down the road.

◆ The Impact on Society

It isn't just senior citizens and low-income families who feel the brunt of high prescription prices. Such prices—and the way they are levied—have an impact on society as a whole. If this can be examined as a public health issue, it's hoped that more can be done to curtail this problem.

The person reading this, who might be fortunate enough to be covered by an employer-backed private insurance plan, might disagree with this assessment. This individual might be paying little to nothing for his or her prescribed drugs, thanks to a low insurance copayment. How on earth could a $10 copay on pharmaceuticals be considered problematic? Furthermore, how can a $10 copay be considered expensive or a burden on society?

This goes back to another economic concept, namely "there ain't no such thing as a free lunch." Even with private insurance covering the cost of high-price drugs (so the individual fortunate to have that type of a plan pays nothing or next to nothing), that cost has to be made up somewhere. The worker might find himself paying slightly higher premiums from one year to the next. Or the employer might find itself shelling over more money to deal with escalating insurance policy costs, in the continued quest to provide health insurance as a benefit to workers. Once upon a time, employer-paid insurance meant few to no deductions taken from paychecks. That is no longer the case. And if insurance premium costs continue increasing, the employer needs to cut something else to pay for it (assuming the employer will even continue offering it, which is another issue). This might mean that the employee might not get a raise for that particular year or overtime might have to be cut.

Furthermore, the complacent individual who pities the senior citizen or lower-income family might be affected in other ways from many of the higher insurance premiums. As mentioned several times in this section, high costs can lead to higher nonadherence to medication. This can be a problem if a disease is contagious. It means that the older person or lower-income individual (or someone who is both of these things) will venture in public, spreading bacterial infections to others. The individual who has a good insurance policy could find himself sitting next to the sick person on a bus or subway and contracting the disease himself. This in turn leads to lost productivity and in some cases could even lead to lost wages. If it's a serious disease such as pneumonia recovery could be a long affair as well.

Nonadherence also leads to higher health care costs down the road, as those who can't afford drugs end up being hospitalized and relying on more expensive treatments. Under the fact that "there ain't no such thing as a free lunch," someone needs to pay for those treatment if the patient can't. More often than not, the "someone" ends up being private insurance companies, who pass on their costs to others in the form of higher premiums. Don't think that government-sponsored insurance is immune either. Those higher costs are going to come out of taxpayers' pockets in the form of higher taxes.

As such, anyone believing that the problem of high drug costs isn't their problem needs to examine how the industry is interrelated. One individual who is nonadherent because she can't afford the price of a drug can end up creating a public health hazard, along with higher societal costs for everyone else. This is why higher drug costs should be considered everyone's problem and not just a problem involving older people or poor people. Unfortunately, to date, drug policy has focused mostly on the how of prescription price coverage. It hasn't yet focused on the why. That focus on the why will be necessary, if there is to be any type of meaningful price reform in this area.

THE ETHICS AND MORALITY OF PHARMACEUTICALS AND PRICES

◆ **Salk and Poliomyelitis**

At the turn of the twentieth century, poliomyelitis was also known as infantile paralysis, and for good reason. Poor sanitation, combined with a misunderstanding of the illness, led to contraction of this disease. The disease struck people of all ages, especially children. Potential effects from the disease ranged from paralysis to difficulty breathing and muscle weakness. While polio wasn't unknown before the mid-twentieth century, it wasn't until post World-War II America that families truly feared polio. At that time, the disease reached epidemic proportions, with the polio outbreak of 1952 being the worst such epidemic in the nation's history. That year, nearly 60,000 were infected with the virus, and more than 3,000 died (Beaubien, 2012). Meanwhile, more than 15,000 cases of paralysis were recorded from the disease (CDC, 2019). If you talk to older people, they will tell you about parks and pools being closed due to fear of contagion. And looking at pictures of polio victims introduces visions of children in "iron lungs" and leg braces, walking with crutches.

Following the introduction of vaccines during the mid-1950s and early 1960s, the number of polio cases in the United States fell to less than one hundred in the 1960s, and fewer than ten by the 1970s (CDC, 2019). The disease in the United States has been all but eradicated today. The killer had been wiped out, thanks to vaccines and Dr. Jonas Salk, who created the "killed-virus" vaccine.

Salk, believing he had a remedy for the problem (and disliking the time it took to develop a live vaccine to treat the disease), proposed a killed-virus vaccine, claiming it would work just as well in "tricking" the body's immune system to fight the disease. This generated a great deal of controversy (live vaccines were the only acceptable solutions for disease mitigation, at the time). Because of the skepticism, Salk tested the killed-virus vaccine on monkeys, then on himself, his wife, and three sons (Klein, 2014). History shows that the vaccine was successful; what followed was the largest experiment in history, funded both by the government and donations from the National Foundation for Infantile Paralysis (today's March of Times). In this experiment, 1.8 million people in the US and Canada signed on to test the drug, through the first-time usage of the double-blind research method. Despite some hiccups, the vaccine was declared to be "safe, effective, and potent" by 1955.

During that same year, legendary newsman Edward R. Murrow interviewed Salk. Murrow asked Salk who owned the patent for the vaccine. Salk's now-famous response was that "the people" owned it, as the research, development and field testing had been funded by charitable donations to the National Foundation for Infantile Paralysis (Duignan, 2013). Because the foundation, a nonprofit organization, had funded it from donations, the vaccine wasn't really in place to make money for anyone. However, when Murrow continued pressing the issue and asking Salk who owned the polio vaccine patent and whether or not there might be a patent, Salk responded, "There is no patent. Could you patent the sun?" (Salk, 1955).

This story is being mentioned not because of the vaccine and eradication of polio (which is a great story, in and of itself) but because Salk's somewhat ambiguous response to Murrow's prodding became the rallying cry of those who decry the huge prices of pharmaceuticals. Those protesting escalating drug prices wave this quote as if shaking a stick, pointing out that drug companies should be in business to provide cures and help people rather than to continue driving profit margins. After all, the argument goes, if Salk's vaccine was offered to the people for no money (and with no patent attached to it), it stands to reason that today's drug companies should be just as altruistic.

This is a somewhat disingenuous response to the issue of higher prescription drug prices, not to mention the issue of whether or not the early polio vaccine should be patented. This is because Salk left some things out of his interview with Murrow. The main omission was that lawyers with the Foundation for Infantile Paralysis did look into the possibility of patenting the vaccine (Smith, 1991). However, the attorneys realized, after researching the issue, that the vaccine didn't meet the so-called "novelty" requirements required for a patent, meaning the application would likely fail and be denied. They didn't want to go through the trouble for a negative response.

Delving into this "novelty" requirement a little more deeply, the question of patents rests on originality of a product, or whether it is unique, with little or no competition. When it comes to vaccines (and patents), there can be questions as to how original they might be, from a development and manufacturing standpoint.

At the time of the Patent Act of 1952, which established the current structure of patent law, there wasn't much recognized difference between "inventions" and "discoveries" (Palmer, 2014). In producing the polio vaccine, Salk didn't so much "invent" it as he discovered it—and discoveries, at the time, were not eligible for patents.

The US Supreme Court attempted to clarify this distinction in 1980, indicating that "products of nature," such as the sun, can't be patented. However, isolating a product, or a molecule of a product, and purifying it could make it eligible for patent. Basically, going back to the basis of pharmaceutical drugs, a poppy flower can't be patented. However, the molecules from that flower, which become opium, can be. This is "discovery" (the poppy flower) versus "invention" (the isolating of the right molecule to make the drug).

Simplifying this, a vaccine might be a product of nature, such as chicken yolks or dead viruses from an animal. Discovering that product, then analyzing it, researching it, and purifying it into a medication is very different from putting the sun to work. Finding the sun is one thing; this is discovery. But taking the light of the sun and through a complicated process bringing it indoors is an invention. The sun can't be patented. However, the device used to channel its light can. According to patent law, there is a difference and distinction between discovery and invention, which wasn't apparent in the 1950s.

Additionally, the decision not to patent the vaccine made good economic sense, not to mention representing a great publicity boon. The foundation funding the research and experimental design of the polio vaccine was a nonprofit organization, as opposed to a for-profit pharmaceutical operation, which it would be expected would collect profits on the sale of a drug or medication. Because the public voluntarily funded the vaccine's very expensive research and testing—through dimes, leading to the March of Dimes slogan and eventual renaming of the organization—it was felt that the public had already paid for the vaccine through its donations. Patenting the vaccine for profit seemed like double charging the public, which is something the foundation's leaders couldn't really stomach (Palmer, 2014).

I've gone into a great deal of discussion about Salk and his vaccine not to paint him as being shady or dishonest about his "patenting the sun" comment. Salk was an intelligent man who accomplished a great deal; thanks to him, children no longer have to fear the ravages of polio. Rather, the discussion is important because there were various legal reasons why the initial vaccine formula wasn't patented. It couldn't be, due to the patent laws at the time.

Needless to say, that's not what we're facing today. Patent requests for drugs today are private corporations. Their goals aren't necessarily 100 percent altruistic. Rather, they invent drugs (notice I don't say "discover" them) to earn profits for themselves and their shareholders. As such, asking these drug manufacturers to forgo patenting their products just because Jonas Salk didn't do so for supposed "altruistic" motives is unreasonable.

Drug companies should be able to earn back what they invest in research on their drugs. They should also be able to earn a good profit on helping society with its ills. The problem occurs, however, when profits and greed override what is right.

◆ The EpiPen Outrage

In the United States, food allergies are considered the leading causes of severe, life-threatening allergic reactions outside of hospitals (ACAAI, 2014). The first line of emergency treatment for anaphylaxis, as it's called, is adrenaline, also known as epinephrine. In recent decades, epinephrine has been available through an auto-injector, which when used correctly immediately reduces airway swelling or low blood pressure that can be common with severe allergy attacks. The hormone involved with the product helps relax muscles, which helps bring almost immediate relief.

Most allergists and doctors recommend that all patients with food allergies (especially children) carry an auto-injector or two in case a severe reaction reoccurs. One of the better-known auto-injectors is marketed under the brand-name EpiPen.

The history of the auto-injector is interesting, as this is not a new product just introduced to the market. EpiPen isn't new either. The former was invented by Sheldon Kaplan as a way to deliver a nerve gas antidote for the US military in the 1970s (Healthline, 2020). And the EpiPen, a version of Kaplan's device, was approved by the FDA in 1987 (Healthline, 2020). The product was far superior to other epinephrine kits at the time as it contained preloaded doses of adrenaline, which could be delivered through a person's clothing. This eliminated the time-consuming process of filling a syringe, not to mention getting rid of the guesswork required to ensure the right dose was being delivered. While Kaplan's name was listed on the device patent, the royalties actually went to his employer, Survival Technology Inc.

From its FDA approval during the late 1980s, the EpiPen changed hands several times over the next twenty years, finally being acquired by pharmaceutical company Mylan in 2007. Mylan didn't really do anything new to or with the drug. Rather, it acquired the right to market the product as part of its overall acquisition of Merck KgA (Healthline, 2020; Miyashiro, 2017).

Within a year of acquiring the EpiPen rights, the company launched a marketing and advocacy campaign, encouraging schools to stock EpiPens in a program called Epi4Schools. The effort was helped by the high-profile deaths of several children from food allergies. President Barack Obama also lent support later on, when in 2013, he signed the School Access to Emergency Epinephrine Act, providing financial incentives to schools for keeping epinephrine auto-injectors on hand.

And because EpiPen had little competition at the time, Mylan thought it was a good idea to increase the prices of this drug and its injector, which had been on the market for more than two decades.

In 2009, a two-pack EpiPen cost $100. This was the wholesale price of the product that pharmacies paid (Miyashiro, 2017). Within a seven-year period, Mylan jacked up the price several times; by 2016, the same two-pack cost $600 (Howard, 2016). This meant that, over a seven-year period, the price of EpiPen had risen by about 500 percent. This was not for a new, blockbuster "specialty" drug geared to treat some narrow disease category. This price increase was for a product that had already been on the market for a long time, which was being used to treat a very large swathe of the population. Much like what happened with Daraprim, there was absolutely no reason or justification for this price increase.

At the same time that Mylan was jacking up the price of EpiPen, it was hiring a lot of lobbyists (Miyashiro, 2017). In addition to using those lobbyists to encourage more states to require epinephrine be made available in public schools, Mylan lobbied the FDA to broaden the wording on the drug's label so that it could be prescribed to those who were "at risk" of anaphylactic shock, in addition to those who had actually experienced it in the past. This effectively broadened the market that could be eligible for this product. By early 2015, Mylan had about 95 percent of the market share, and in 2016, Mylan exceeded a billion dollars in EpiPen sales. This was the same year during which the $600 price tag drew widespread criticism from the public as well as intense scrutiny from lawmakers. Congressional committees requested that Mylan explain the price increases, with the end result being a hearing by the House Committee on Oversight and Government Reform in September 2016.

During the hearing, Heather Bresch, who had been CEO of Mylan since 2011, faced a great deal of criticism during her testimony; she was unable to specifically answer questions about revenues or patient assistance programs (Miyashiro, 2017). She did, however, defend her company's business practices and refused to admit that the company had raised the price of EpiPens to increase corporate profits (Miyashiro, 2017). She pointed out that the price surge was due to increased research and development costs as well as the school program. Remember the "increase research and development" might be somewhat questionable as the product itself didn't change at all. She claimed that half of the wholesale price of EpiPen was received by insurance companies and pharmacy benefit managers. In other words, Bresch pointed the finger of blame elsewhere other than herself, at a "broken" health care system (Egan (b), 2016). Apparently, she felt that she could take advantage of such a system.

It was somewhat difficult to sympathize with Bresch's predicament, especially when it was reported that she had earned $19 million in total compensation in 2015 (Egan, 2016). The American Medical Association didn't buy her argument either, pointing out that the product had been unchanged since 2009 (Egan, 2016). The AMA also pointed out that the higher price threatened to keep EpiPens out of the reach of people who might need it or to force families to cut back on other essentials to pay for the medication (Egan, 2016).

The EpiPen scandal differed from that of Daraprim. While the situation with Daraprim was bad, the high cost of the EpiPen affected a larger population, with a more common ailment: food allergies. Furthermore, the obscenely high price was affecting families with children, whose only fault was that they might have unknowingly ingested a little peanut butter with their airways swelling closed as a result. In other words, the lack of an EpiPen on hand, due to the high price tag, could conceivably kill a child. This, in fact, was what Mylan was demonstrating when pushing more EpiPens into schools through its EpiPen4Schools program.

Finally, public backlash against Mylan and CEO Bresch was huge and more pronounced than what happened with the Pharma Bro and his Daraprim. Outraged parents and others took to social media to shame Mylan for the price increase (Egan (b), 2016). And in the face of the backlash, Mylan announced it would take steps to reduce the costs, partly by introducing a generic EpiPen and partly by providing patients with instant savings cards (Howard, 2016).

However, this didn't prevent lawsuits from being filed against Mylan in response to issues such as classification of EpiPen as a "generic" drug (in an effort to avoid higher rebates that are required to be paid for the sale of brand-name drugs to state Medicaid programs). Another lawsuit involved an antitrust investigation, in that sales contracts with schools as part of the EpiPen4Schools program violated antitrust laws. Still more lawsuits charged Mylan with illegal schemes to dominate the market with PBMs and illegally attempting to prevent competition for the EpiPen. A lack of competition also meant that Mylan could continue to increase prices for the product.

Despite all of those lawsuits, EpiPen is still being sold, and Mylan is still in business, churning out their product for a fair amount of money. In other words, nothing much has changed, despite the public outrage, congressional inquiries, and legal challenges.

There is no doubt that Mylan, or any other pharmaceutical company, for that matter, should be allowed to charge what the market can bear for a product. But did Mylan (and CEO Bresch) go beyond the issue of ethical behavior by increasing the cost of the drug by 500 percent?

Sweeping aside the emotion and response generated by Mylan's somewhat unorthodox pricing practices, Vendavo pricing consultant Daniel Kozarich (2016) compared Mylan's price-raising strategy to a five-step "price ethics" test listed in the book *The Strategy and Tactics of Pricing: A Guide to Growing More Profitably* (Nagle, Hogan and Zale, 2016).

According to Kozarich, Mylan seemed to pass ethical test number 1, in which the buyer of a product knows the price and voluntarily completes the transaction (Kozarich, 2016; Nagle, Hogan and Zale, 2016). There was nothing opaque about the $600 EpiPen price; most people knew about it and, for whatever reasons, were willing to pay that price rather than go without the drug's benefits. Certainly, complaints were lodged. But in the end, most voluntarily completed the transactions, even knowing the price.

Mylan also passed the second ethical price test in that it didn't mislead consumers in terms of price or quality. Again, the price was well-known. There was nothing hidden about it so people couldn't say later on that they'd been duped. The same thing could be said with ethical pricing test number 5, in which the exchange presented equal access to goods (Kozarich, 2016; Nagle, Hogan and Zale, 2016). Mylan passed this ethical test as well. Consumers did have access to discounts, based on financial need. Additionally, Mylan provided free EpiPens to schools (and continues to do so). This does provide the indication that if a student should suffer an anaphylaxis attack, he or she will have access to the necessary medication to ensure that such an attack won't have any long-term consequences.

Where Mylan miserably failed its pricing ethics through the ethics' list points three and four. The third test indicated that sellers can't exploit a buyer's essential needs, while test number four points out that price must be justified by costs (Kozarich, 2016; Nagle, Hogan and Zale, 2016).

Let's look at these. Mylan prevented competition from entering the field through antitrust activities, thus meaning that EpiPen was the only game in town when it came to treatment of anaphylactic shock. Basically, it seems as though antitrust behaviors were the only way in which Mylan could continue generating any kind of profit on the drug. The patent protection had expired, but there was still consistent demand, both due to need and due to the one-year shelf life. As such, the company was able to create a monopoly in which it could set its own price. The only choice the consumer had was to go without and save the $600 price (assuming insurance wouldn't cover this) or risk death from an allergic reaction.

This also brings us to the failure the fourth test, that of price being justified by costs. Increasing the EpiPen price from $100 to more than $600 over a six-year period went well beyond cost justifications. Certainly, the EpiPen4Schools program would cost a bit. No one would deny that ensuring product availability in schools would require a capital investment. However, it was Mylan that initiated and drove the program not because of altruism but to obtain contracts from schools and to broaden its market share. The schools didn't approach Mylan for the drug; Mylan deliberately, and systematically, set up the campaign to get the schools on board. Additionally, increasing the price of the product from $300 to $600 over a two-year period boosted Mylan's profit margin as high as 55 percent (Kozarich, 2016). Commented Kozarich, "There should be no excessive, unjustified profits on essentials." A 55 percent profit margin could be considered both excessive and unjustified. It's for these reasons that Mylan's behavior moves from a pharmaceutical company that is trying to make profits for shareholders into one that is behaving in a very unethical fashion.

According to Wells Fargo analyst David Maris,

No one's expecting Mylan to give away their products. But empathy is the most human emotion. And
when you raise the price year after year ... for a drug
that's lifesaving, it shows a complete lack of empathy.
(Egan (b), 2016)

While Mylan and EpiPen represent probably the most egregious
and unethical behavior by a pharmaceutical company to the public
it is supposed to serve, it is not, by far, the only one to operate in
such a fashion. If it hasn't been guessed by now, the pharmaceutical
industry doesn't do a very good job behaving in an ethical fashion,
an inability to "patent the sun" notwithstanding.

◆ Ethical Myopia

Two years after Mylan ran afoul of public, Congress, and terrible
PR, *Forbes* contributor Robert Pearl was waiting for a plane at Dulles
Airport, where he logged onto the internet and found a story about
Nirmal Mulye, CEO of Nostrum Laboratories. Mulye was explaining why he'd raised the price of an antibiotic drug, nitrofurantoin,
from less than $500 to more than $2,000 (Pearl, 2018). The reason,
apparently, was because "I think it's a moral requirement to make
money when you can," Mulye had said, comparing his pricing strategy to that of an art dealer who sells a painting for a half a billion
dollars (Pearl, 2018). Once again, nitrofurantoin was not a blockbuster specialty drug developed to cure a rare form of cancer or a
painful form of rheumatoid arthritis. Rather, it is a liquid antibiotic
that has been on the market since the early 1950s. Liquid antibiotics

are typically given to people who find it difficult to take pills, such as children or the elderly (Crow, 2018). They do cost more to manufacture as they are more complicated to make (Crow, 2018).

However, the only justification for the price increase on this particular product was due to supply shortages of the liquid version. This in turn had been prompted by new rules on impurities, under the auspices of the FDA. So in this case, the regulations were the catalyst; Nostrum did have to pull the product from the market to have it conform to FDA regulations (and it probably wouldn't be surprising if the company took out a new patent on it). But it's uncertain as to whether this justifies a 400 percent price increase on a drug, expensive paintings and out-of-touch pricing strategies notwithstanding (Pearl, 2018).

Pear's observations on Mulye's comments were that, first of all, an art dealer who sells a painting for a lot of money can do so because those who might be interested in buying such a painting have a choice. They can pay the money for the painting and walk away with it or pay nothing. Their lives won't change whether they own that painting or not, unless they are obsessive art connoisseurs, of course.

But pharmaceuticals and drugs are different from a luxury item like a painting. Patients who are often in need of drugs don't have much of a choice about it. If they go without a drug, they'll become sicker and their quality of life will diminish. In the case of the liquid nitrofurantoin, this is especially apparent, given its "target audience" of elderly people and children. While there are plenty of antibiotics on the market, those that are in liquid form are limited. In a sense, such a price increase can make affordability difficult.

As such, if an elderly person or the family of a child puts money

toward the huge costs of a drug—even something like nitrofurantoin, they have to sacrifice something else, like food or even rent. As
a result, patients in need often don't have the ability to buy that drug.
Already, "many Americans are suffering the consequences of rising
drug prices," Pearl noted. In this case, Mulye and his company fail
ethical tests three and four, much as Bresch did in the case of Mylan
(Nagle, Hogan and Zale, 2016). The difference, however, is that
Mulye owns his beliefs, as distasteful, out of touch, and unethical as
they are. Bresch didn't even have the dignity to take responsibility
for the profits and price increases.

Back to the nitrofurantoin price increase. Despite the fact that it
was the FDA that (indirectly) led to the price increase—it was said
that Nostrum had to remove its version of nitrofurantoin from the
market to reformulate it to comply with the new regulations—it was
somewhat ironic that criticism for the price hike came from FDA
commissioner Scott Gottlieb. He pointed out,

> There is no moral imperative to price gouge and take
> advantage of patients. FDA will continue to promote
> competition so speculators and those with no regard
> to public health consequences can't take advantage
> of patients who need medicine. (Crow, 2018)

Mulye's response was that the FDA was "incompetent and cor-
rupt," with the new rules on impurities as a "piece of nonsense"
(Crow, 2018).

Whether the FDA was justified or not in its new "impurities"
rule isn't really at issue. What is at issue is that not only did Nostrum

Laboratories increase the price of a drug but its CEO owned that decision, suggesting that it was OK to charge as much as possible for a sixty-year-old drug that is given to elderly people and children. Specifically, the CEO deliberately understood his actions would increase the price, making it more expensive for a select market to be able to afford the drug. This is not an ethical action. This is a greedy action, performed by a pharmaceutical executive, just because he can.

◆ Affordability and Availability

One crux involving drug prices focuses on their affordability. It's been established throughout this book (and will continue to be established) that pharmaceuticals in the United States are not very affordable. As a result, not everyone who needs the drugs can have access to them, depending on their income, type of drug, where it is sold, how it is sold, or even what kind of insurance plan an individual might be on.

But what is a "just" price for a drug, or any good, for that matter? What is considered "ethical pricing," in this case? The likely, ethical answer to these questions is that the price for a drug should be such that maintains a reasonable profit to drug companies, while being fair, accessible, and affordable to patients and the health care system (Kantarjian, Steensma, Sanjuan, Elshaug, and Light, 2014). Right now, we don't know if drug prices are just, according to this definition of ethics, because we actually don't know how much a manufacturer's list price is on various drugs—unless such a list price is publicized. Certainly, we know the costs of EpiPen, Daraprim, and nitrofurantoin.

But we don't know how much it costs to manufacture or market these drugs, thereby making it difficult to determine if the price provides a reasonable profit to the companies. The chances are good that the answer is the price provides well above a reasonable profit.

And this explanation as to just pricing and ethics would make sense, if pharma manufacturers and consumers were the only stakeholders involved with the buying and selling of drugs. Along those lines, Big Pharma is bad enough when it comes to fair pricing. While there is merit that the cost of researching, manufacturing, and distributing drugs can be quite high, there is also merit to the idea that these drug companies are charging high prices for drugs, both without transparency and without justification for the price increases.

Big Pharma's pricing activities are worsened by the fact that that determining the actual value of a drug and determining "fair" pricing differs along the drug supply chain.

It's worth repeating that the drug supply chain has many stakeholders, all of which have a hand in product pricing (Alvaro, Challener, and Branch, 2019). The manufacturer must estimate the size of the market of the drug, in relationship to the cost of the drug's development. PBMs also like to be paid through their "rebates," which can have an impact on drug pricing. Furthermore, before determining a specific price, a pharmaceutical company will consult with insurance companies to determine what their direct competitors are charging. The price of a new drug that performs better than a previously marketed treatment can be increased by a 10 percent-15 percent markup, on average. This is why Gilead's Sovaldi, a hepatitis C treatment, entered the market with a $84,000 price tag, higher than existing hep C therapies. Was this an ethical pricing decision? Again, this is hard to say, given we don't know all of the costs involved with the drug. Nor can we examine this question in light of the benefits, which involve a potential lowering of costs down the road, in the form of a potential liver transplant. The "ethics" here could be that a patient is paying that high price, in order to avoid a $500,000 price tag for a new liver. This could, in a strange way, be considered "ethical."

Insurance companies, meanwhile, are the ones on the front lines of combatting drug prices. They set budgets for the year in advance, before even knowing what drugs will be offered or at what cost. These companies have internal measures to keep costs low, such as prior authorizations or making a patient take part in a so-called "step therapy" system. Through such a system, the patient is required to try other drugs before a more costly therapy can be prescribed. But in some cases, insurance companies don't always behave ethically either. More of the cost sharing of prescriptions is being put on the patient. But again, without knowing what the company's actual costs are, we don't really know if those costs are "just." It might not seem like it, especially when public insurance companies are required to report their profits.

The end result here is that the patient—the ultimate consumer of the drug—has little to no input when it comes to the pricing process. Rather, patients are squeezed between insurance companies and drug companies (with PBMs throw in for good measure), none of which are being held accountable for consumer interests. This is actually the real ethical problem that consumer interests aren't being looked after.

There is an inherent conflict between the desire (and need) for affordable drugs and expectations and obligations to shareholders and other investors in pharmaceutical companies for a competitive return on investment. But as it currently stands, different patients pay different prices for the exact same drug, with prices based on specifics of their health insurance plans, geographic location, and even where that drug is acquired. And unless we truly understand the costs of manufacturing and getting these drugs to market, it's impossible to determine the ethics behind such decisions.

◆ Ethics versus Profit

The American public has gotten used to the argument that it's impossible to be a fully ethical company while making a profit for shareholders. This is because implementation of ethics (such as good environmental practices, getting rid of animal testing, or not charging an arm and a leg for drugs), will cost more money. It will reduce profit margins, putting corporations into the poor house, laying off thousands of people, and so on. What these protesting companies don't seem to realize is that other corporations have been able to incorporate ethical practices and still earn decent profits. But it's easier not to put the money into ethical behavior; doing so does require an investment of time, consideration, and yes, monies.

But ethics isn't a black-or-white issue. An organization doesn't have to operate solely on solar power and wind turbines to be an ethical one. By the same token, pharmaceutical organizations don't have to cut their profits to the bare bones to be considered ethical. No one is suggesting that such companies don't have a right to make a profit on patents or products.

But pharmaceutical companies, as are health care organizations in general, are in a tricky position. They are responsible for seeing to the well-being of a society, in addition to making money on products and services. This puts pharmaceutical manufacturers (at least in their minds) in the crosshairs of profit versus ethics. The problem comes about when such organizations make decisions in which profit trumps ethics and then claim it is OK because a pharmaceutical company should take as much as it can, while it can.

When it comes to ethical issues in health care (including pharmaceuticals), there are four bioethical principles: beneficence, nonmaleficence, autonomy, and justice (Drettwan and Kjos, 2019). Additionally, some pharmaceutical texts focus on fidelity and truthfulness as more recent ethical principles.

How do these compare to theoretical ethical models? Let's take a look at some of the more common ethical models.

- The utility model (also known as utilitarianism) maximizes good for a society while minimizing harm.
- The exceptions model focuses on the ethical nature if an individual exception becomes the standard norm for all.
- The choices model focuses on how decisions are made, with the emphasis placed on moral respect for individual choices.
- The justice model considers limited resources distribution, pointing out that resources should be distributed to areas where they will do the most good.
- The common good model, similar to the utility model, focuses on how decisions might benefit everyone, as opposed to a single individual.
- The virtue model emphasizes core values aspired to by the decider, determining whether a given scenario might help or hinder someone when it comes to reaching those values.

When analyzing the above ethical models against both the Pharmacist Code of Ethics and the Physician Code of Ethics, Drettwan and Kjos (2019) found that behavior of PBMs, for example, were highly unethical, as indicated in the chart below.

Scenario and Model	Market Consolidation	Pharmacy Reimbursement Rate	Gag Clauses	Exclusion Lists	Point of Sale Rebates	Totals
Utility	Ethical	Unethical	Ethical	Ethical	Ethical	Ethical: 4 Unethical: 1
Exceptions	Unethical	Unethical	Ethical	Ethical	Unethical	Ethical: 2 Unethical: 3
Choices	Unethical	Unethical	Unethical	Unethical	Ethical	Ethical: 1 Unethical: 4
Justice	Unethical	Unethical	Unethical	Ethical	Ethical	Ethical: 2 Unethical: 3
Common Good	Unethical	Unethical	Unethical	Unethical	Ethical	Ethical: 4 Unethical: 1
Virtue	Ethical	Unethical	Unethical	Unethical	Ethical	Ethical: 1 Unethical: 4
Pharmacist	Unethical	Unethical	Unethical	Unethical	Ethical	Ethical: 2 Unethical: 2
Physician	Unethical	Unethical	N/A	Ethical	Ethical	Ethical: 2 Unethical: 2
Totals	Ethical: 2 Unethical: 6	Ethical: 0 Unethical: 8	Ethical: 2 Unethical: 5	Ethical: 4 Unethical: 4	Ethical: 7 Unethical: 1	Ethical: 15/39 Unethical: 24/39

However, the current way in which the US pharmaceutical industry is structured leads to conflicting interests, one of which is making drugs affordable from the standpoint of patients and society versus making new drugs available from research and development efforts.

Delving into this more deeply, affordability is defined as how easy, or feasible, an individual (or society) finds it to pay for a drug, and it is a function of prices, insurance coverage, a family's financial circumstances, and to an extent, the drug's purpose. As an example, $200 might be considered too expensive for a drug to prevent migraine headaches. However, $200 might not be too expensive to save, or prolong, a person's life. Meanwhile, availability focuses on the presence or absence of particular types of drugs in the marketplace. The problem we run into with pharmaceuticals is that sometimes availability can affect affordability. And when affordability comes into question, it can lead to serious societal problems.

◆ Pricier than Gold

Let's look at the story of yet another hugely priced drug. In 2019, and with the blessing of the FDA, Zolgensma, manufactured by Novartis, became the world's priciest prescription medication (Pearl, 2019). The drug, a one-dose gene therapy geared to cure children with spinal muscular atrophy, was priced at $2.125 million per patient (Pearl, 2019). The problem here is that an independent assessment actually priced the drug at up to $900,000 per patient; while a large sum, this is one-fifth the price that Novartis is commanding for selling the product. Needless to say, the huge price of this treatment focused on the rights of Novartis and other pharmaceutical companies to price "orphan drugs"—those that are released for rare diseases—at what the market will bear.

This could probably have been viewed through a more ethical lens overall, had Novartis actually put resources into inventing, researching, and going through clinical trials of the drug. But Novartis didn't do any of this. Rather, it acquired AveXis, the firm that did invent, research, and clinically test the drug (Pearl, 2019). Given the price tag of the drug, Novartis will recoup the acquisition costs in relative short order (Pearl, 2019; Campbell, 2019). In this case, the cost of the drug very much outweighs the justified price, at least according to the pricing ethics test. Yet the outrage and cries of ethical foul were not nearly as extreme when it came to this price tag, at least not as compared to Daraprim and EpiPen. Why is this?

For one thing, the drug is vastly different from both pharmaceuticals and even biologics. It is not a pharmaceutical so much as it is gene therapy. In fact it's the second gene therapy that has been FDA approved. It is a very new drug, which might lead one to assume that Novartis is still taking a risk in offering it as a treatment. It is also used to treat "truly sick patients" (Campbell, 2019). Second, the convenience factor, combined with the power of the drug, means it is actually less expensive, overall, than its nearest competition, Spinraza. This actually goes back to the Sovaldi story, in which the expense of the treatment now could help prevent even more horrifying or expensive treatments down the road.

Furthermore, the beneficiaries of Zolgensma—the parents of children with SMA—indicate that putting a price on a child's life isn't something they want to do (Pearl, 2019). These parents are concerned that if drug manufacturers such as Novartis aren't allowed to make their profits off drugs such as Zolgensma, there would be little to any incentive to cure orphan diseases. To these parents, the price is "just" because it guarantees survival and better quality of life for their children.

All of this would be acceptable—if it weren't for the pricing strategy tests introduced by *The Strategy and Tactics of Pricing: A Guide to Growing More Profitably*. Certainly, gene therapy is pricey to research and implement. But the ethical problem here is that Novartis did nothing to create this drug. Rather, the company bought the company that had spent all the money researching and developing Zolgensma. Basically, it is making a profit on an acquisition, not recouping vast millions spent on creating this product. Yes, it treats "very sick children." And yes, in a sense, it is less expensive than its nearest competition. And yes, the consumer believes the price is worth the results and is willing to pay that price. But from an ethical standpoint, Novartis's behavior doesn't measure up to the situation. Novartis didn't buy AveXis because it wanted to help distribute a drug to help society. It bought the company so it could reap profits on an insanely expensive treatment for a rare disease.

In this case, "intent" is probably more the driver of whether this is an ethical decision or not. How do we know it's not ethical? Because of the fact that, to recoup its costs and earn a decent profit, Novartis only had to charge $900,000. Instead, it chose to drive the price up to more than $2 million. Orphan drug or not, this seems a bit excessive, even for all the good this drug is likely to do.

This is where ethics and pharmaceutical companies don't seem to match. Criteria guiding drug company R&D decisions isn't so much the moral good or societal considerations as much as it rests on profits. Specifically, drug companies don't consider what will best benefit society, then plan to make money off of that. Rather, these companies begin by determining which treatments are the most likely to command high prices and to turn fast profits. The treatment for SMA fulfills both of these requirements.

Next, drug manufacturers seek out captive audiences, assessing the needs and motivations of at-risk populations while calculating the likelihood of gaining insurance reimbursements. When it comes to SMA, which is quickly diagnosed and fatal, again, this fits the requirement. And finally, these drugmakers seek out solutions with minimum upfront investments, such as Novartis bypassing expensive R&D costs by purchasing the drug's developer for $8.7 billion.

Finally, there is the focus on what will be a guaranteed slam-dunk for profits versus what is likely to be of benefit. Zolgensma will clearly be a slam-dunk involving treatment for a very painful and debilitating disease.

But in another example, glioblastoma multiforme (GBM) is a brain cancer with a very high fatality rate and horrible prognosis. It's actually a fairly well-known and publicized disease. Edward Kennedy, US senator from Massachusetts, had it and brought awareness to the condition (Sorter, 2013). More recently, Senator John McCain died from the same disease. While interest has grown in the research of the disease itself, it hasn't had much input from the pharmaceutical industry namely because "it is a fairly uncommon cancer. We might see about 10,000 cases in the US every year," Manmeet Ahluwalia, staff physician at the Rose Ella Burkhardt Brain Tumor & Neuro-Oncology Center at the Cleveland Clinic in Ohio, told *Cure Today Magazine*. While 10,000 might seem to be a lot of patients in a given year, it's apparently not cost-effective for pharmaceutical companies to treat this horrific, and almost always fatal disease, even with two high-profile senators having it. What is more cost-effective, it seems, is treating the millions of men who have erectile dysfunction or having multiple different brands of high-priced insulin available. In this case, ethics seems to be taking a serious back seat.

◆ Profits versus Ethics: Mutually Exclusive?

Due to drug life cycle dynamics (and yes, the expense involved with manufacturing), the main strategy of drug companies is to increase prices to maintain high revenues, whenever and however they can (van der Gronde, Uyl-de Groot, and Pieters, 2017). As such, the top ten pharmaceutical companies have a profit margin of 20 percent on average; those in the S&P 1500 have a net profit margin of 16 percent, compared to 7 percent for all other companies in the index. This is because higher drug prices compensate for lower product turnover while protecting the high-profit profile. Is this excessive? Again, a 20 percent profit margin on a product could be considered somewhat excessive, especially if such a number comes at the expense of providing society with what it needs. Though this process of continually increasing prices for little justifiable reason helps drug companies continue to keep shareholders happy, it does mean it doesn't benefit society as a whole. This is also a good example of how "just" pricing seems to take a dive.

This is especially the case when prices skyrocket on pharmaceuticals that have been on the market for not just years but decades. In these situations, the drug has been around long enough for it to become a staple in patients' lives. They depend on that drug for survival and quality of life. But when a higher price threatens access to such a drug for no good reason (other than the fact that "we can do it"), it suggests a horrific breach of ethics. Adding to the difficulty is that poor ethics won't put pharmaceutical executives into jail, nor will it encourage any kind of accountability. Pharma Bro Martin Shkreli was sent to prison not because he raised the price on a drug by 400 percent but because of securities fraud related to his company. That apparently was illegal, while monopolistic price increases were not. Mylan's former CEO, Heather Bresch, was never jailed for her role in EpiPen's price increase. In fact, she is helping to direct the merger between Mylan and Pfizer's Upjohn Unit, from which she'll collect a cool $37.6 million when she retires, following the close of the sale (Sagonowksy, 2019). Nor is Nirmal Mulye with Nostrum Laboratories facing more than a media lashing and verbal lashings from the FDA. He remains secure in the belief that it's OK to charge what the market will bear.

In a way, he isn't wrong. The very basis of capitalism is to price a product in line with demand. But Big Pharma has a double responsibility, both to its shareholders and the general public. With its pricing policies, and actions of other stakeholders, from PBMs to pharmacists, there is no sense of responsibility to the public.

Again, as I keep reiterating, there is absolutely nothing shameful about making a profit on a product, even if that product is a drug. Profits are justified; they keep American companies running and able to produce more products. Nor is there anything illegal about increasing the price of drugs to stratospheric levels. From a moral standpoint, it's repugnant, especially when the company doing so has responsibility to the public for health and welfare. But Big Pharma, along with PBMs and insurance companies, doesn't seem to care. They acknowledge that prices have gotten out of control, but rather than coming together and figuring out ways to deal with it all, the response is blaming and finger-pointing. Meanwhile, all of the media-shaming, protests, and even complaints from Washington policymakers have no impact on this industry. We know this because the high prices keep happening. The only thing that can help start keeping prices in check is to take note of what other countries are doing to control higher drug prices and to follow suit.

US VERSUS THE WORLD: COMPARING PHARMACEUTICAL PRICES

IN HIS 2005 BOOK *A CALL TO ACTION: TAKING BACK Healthcare for Future Generations,* author Hank McKinnell (who was, at the time, chairman and CEO of Pfizer Inc.) attempted to tackle the problem of drug prices. Specifically, his focus was why branded drugs were less expensive in Canada than the United States. His answer to this comparison was "The Canadian government caps the amount that US pharmaceutical companies can charge Canadian pharmacies, distributors, and wholesalers" (p. 63).

After this honest assessment and commentary, McKinnell then demonstrates that the Canadian government is apparently the real villain when it comes to lower pharmaceutical prices, pointing out that

> once pharmaceutical companies have sunk the re-
> search costs necessary to develop medicines, govern-
> ments often use their powers as regulators, dominant

purchasers and arbiters of intellectual property
rights to enforce their demands. (p. 64)

McKinnell goes on to suggest that poor, misunderstood pharmaceutical companies such as Pfizer are unable to fight sovereign nations, especially those nations that dare to supply local manufacturers to produce a drug, should "free-market prices" (as he calls them) become too high.

Clearly, he is no fan of price controls. He goes into a great deal of commentary about the dangers of price controls and subsidies (ignoring the fact that PBM rebates are, in themselves, a form of subsidizing by pharmaceutical manufacturers). Sure, he makes a decent argument that de facto price controls can stifle innovation in new drugs. No one is really disputing this. The question he fails to answer in his diatribe, however, is whether we really need those new treatments or "blockbuster drugs" that Pfizer and its competition keeps trundling out. The US seems to think so because its system is set up to reward these blockbuster drugs. Foreign governments, on the other hand, don't think that all the blockbuster drugs churned out by these companies are necessary. Their pharmaceutical approval agencies and authorities actually don't approve blockbuster drugs, unless there is a good reason to do so (Sarnak, Squares, Kuzmak and Bishop, 2017).

For the most part, other countries will assess a few things when considering approval of a new drug. They will focus on not just the effectiveness of a new drug but whether that particular drug is more effective than existing therapies and, in some cases, whether it is even more cost-effective than what is already being offered in the marketplace. As such, while per-person drug utilization in the US matches that of other countries, research indicates that the mix of drugs consumed in the United States includes a higher proportion of newer, more expensive medicines but no clear evidence as to better outcomes (Sarnak, Squires, and Bishop, 2017).

Additionally, the centralized price-control negotiations employed in different countries involve national formularies and comparative cost-effectiveness research for determining price ceilings. This is in direct contrast to US methods, which are more of a free-for-all in which any drug price is fair game. Furthermore, the US permits "wider latitude for monopoly pricing of brand-name drugs than other countries are willing to accept." And unlike the FDA in the United States, similar organizations in other countries are more willing to compare efficacy between the "new drug" and other drugs already on the market before issuing approval for the newer version.

For a pharmaceutical company that is interested in boosting the price of a particular drug, such price controls and approval processes can be annoying. It's no wonder Mr. McKinnell turns his nose up at Canadian pharmaceutical pricing policies.

◆ Pharmaceuticals by the Numbers

According to the most recent data from OCED, the United States spending per capita on pharmaceuticals was $1,221 (OCED, 2019). We know this is a high rate, especially as the next-highest national spending was Switzerland, which came in at $894 per capita.

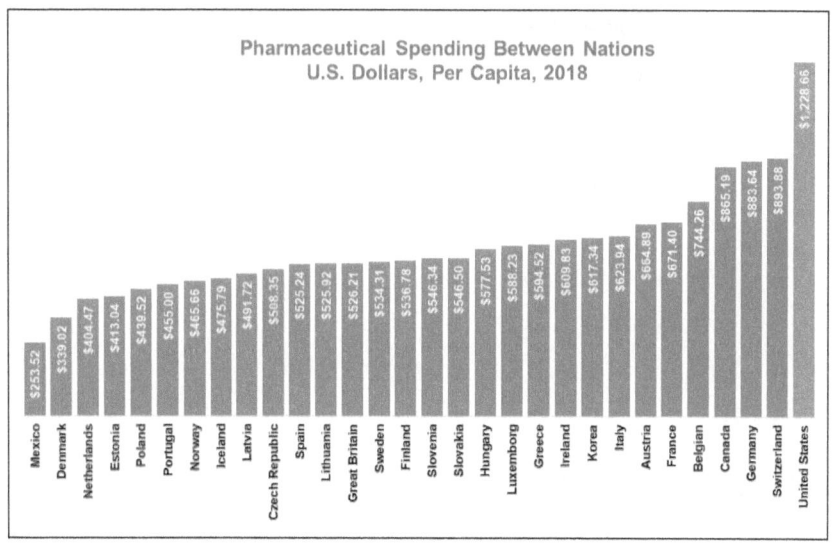

Pharmaceutical Spending Between Nations
U.S. Dollars, Per Capita, 2018

Though we've focused on monopolistic practices and other factors as main reasons why US patients pay so much in prescription drugs, the question ends up being how it is that competing nations can get away with lower prices. This question is especially pertinent as Sarnak et al. (2017) pointed out that during the 1980s, "several countries spent about the same amount per capita as the US."

Yet we already know what happened during the last decade of the twentieth century: the ramp-up of "blockbuster drug" releases, with sales of both hypertensive and cancer drugs booming (Sarnak, Squires, and Bishop, 2017). Added to this was expansions of insurance coverage—including those of prescription drugs—by the federal government through Medicare, Medicaid, and the Children's Health Insurance Program (CHIPS).

To put this into the realm of research, Sarnak and his colleagues, in their 2017 brief for the Commonwealth Fund, indicated four potential factors that determine a country's spending on pharmaceuticals:

- country population and volume of drugs consumed
- drug utilization per person
- type and mix of drugs consumed (as in genetics versus brand-name drugs)
- prices at which drugs are sold

To play fair, the US does have the largest population and greatest absolute prescription drug spending as a country. Basically, we're bigger than everyone else in the world. However, even with these factors in mind, the US spending per capita on pharmaceuticals is "still significantly higher than that of other countries." It's not even that Americans are popping more pills than their international counterparts. They aren't. Drug utilization in the US is not significantly higher than that of other countries (Sarnak, Squires, and Bishop, 2017). What is significantly higher in the US versus the world is drug prices overall, especially prices of blockbuster drugs. The reason for this, as McKinnell disingenuously pointed out, is that other countries do much more than the US to limit patient exposure to higher, out-of-pocket costs, implementing caps at certain price levels.

But this is not the problem just of pharmaceuticals. Out-of-control prices are a problem of the US health care system as a whole, and the US has struggled to control these for similar reasons— namely, the wrong things are being targeted when it comes to health care reform. Other nations do a much better job of limiting overall out-of-pocket costs for health care. In fact, health care delivery and payment systems in other countries are far less fragmented than they are in the United States; this fragmentation adds administrative and other cost burdens to the problem. This means Americans overall are forced to bear higher costs because the US is the only industrialized country with a large, uninsured population, even after passage of the Affordable Healthcare Act. Additionally, even Americans who carry health insurance—even decent health insurance, backed by their employers—tend to have fewer protective benefits than their counterparts in other nations. Finally, due to escalating health prices, the solution seems to be that consumers should coshare costs, rather than taking the time and putting resources toward why these costs are becoming so high in the first place.

Combining this with the lack of price control strategies and fragmented nature of the overall health care system puts the US at a high cost per capita of pharmaceuticals, especially when compared to Canada, Germany, or the United Kingdom. The lack of central negotiating power that McKinnell derides so much also makes drugs more expensive—and this has nothing to do with research or development. Rather, it boils down to the fact that each private payer has to negotiate separately for prices on drugs with each manufacturer, rather than leaving it to one centralized entity. Added to this fragmented way of determining prices, additional complex arrangements for payments and pricing are put into place among various federal and state health programs, such as Medicare and Medicaid. And this bears repeating: Medicare is not allowed to negotiate directly with drug manufacturers for reduced prices, which is a problem. The end result continues to be escalating prices, especially due to administrative burdens of continuing to sustain the United States' ever-growing unwieldy health care system.

◆ Baskets of Drugs

Other developed nations (*not* the United States) protect consumers from increasing drug prices by using an external reference pricing system also known as ERP (House Committee on Ways and Means, 2019). An ERP system uses the price of a pharmaceutical product in one or several countries to formulate a benchmark, or reference price, against which to set or negotiate pharmaceutical prices in a given country. Almost every European country—Denmark, Sweden, and the United Kingdom excepted—has some form of ERP. Most other developed nations also have some kind of established ERP in place. This helps determine what is fair pricing versus prices that are out of control. This is also a transparent system in that just about everyone knows the "real" cost of a particular drug, rather than an estimated cost. Understanding the real cost of a drug, when it is first manufactured, can help when it comes to comparisons and decent pricing.

To develop their ERPs, these countries create a "basket" of drug rates in comparable countries and use the average of all prices in that basket as a benchmark from which to determine fair pricing practices. The United States could do this too, as long as it had a central agency charged with researching and averaging comparable drug prices across Canada, Australia, the United Kingdom, and Ireland, as an example of English-speaking countries only. (It could throw Europe in for good measure if it wanted to.) Then, once this central authority had an average benchmark, it could go back to the pharmaceutical companies and point out that prices being charged for certain drugs in the US are higher than that basket average. Then, backed by legislation, it could force the companies to do something about the higher prices.

Incidentally, when it comes to averaging and negotiating drugs, most countries don't bother with entities, such as pharmaceutical benefit managers or private insurance companies, and the extra prices they might charge. Rather, they will use the actual manufacturer prices—in other words, the prices that the pharma maker charges wholesalers or pharmacies—for ERPs. There are some differences, of course. For example, Finland relies on wholesale prices for its comparisons, while the Netherlands will rely on retail prices.

Furthermore, every country relying on an ERP uses publicly available price information. In other words, rather than being shrouded in secrecy due to gag orders, confidential discounts, and opaque rebate amounts negotiated between payers, PBMS, and manufacturers, these countries have a transparent, public list from which they can obtain prices. It is the United States that continues to remain in the dark as to what drugs actually cost.

Does this "drug basket" work? Empirical evidence suggests that the answer is yes. One study showed that ERP methods led to reductions in drug prices of about 15 percent over a ten-year period (Panteli, et al., 2016). As such, this is something that might be worth a try to keep a handle on drug prices. The problem is the McKinnells of the world would likely not accept this.

◆ Moving Internally

In addition to very global and very public comparisons of drug rates, countries that are *not* the United States also make use of an internal reference price (IRP), which is typically used in pricing generic drugs. The IRPs help determine fair drug prices, based on market equivalents or similar products already within the country (House Committee on Ways and Means, 2019; Panteli et al., 2016). They are also used to set payment rates for product groups that cluster drugs according to active substance or therapeutic class.

So if for fun we were to examine market equivalents of erectile dysfunction drugs in the United States (based on manufacturers price of brand-name drugs), an IRP would focus on pinpointing fair drug prices for their generic equivalent. Using an IRP might not get rid of issues such as reverse payments or "pay for delay." That will have to be up to the government to work through that one, as will be indicated later on in this paper. But an IRP can ensure that once they are released to the market, generic drugs will be priced in a fair, competitive, and ethical manner.

The issue here, of course, is that pharmaceutical manufacturers would need to be willing to release the actual, base price for their drugs and that the price be a "just" one—in other words, enough to cover the basic costs of research, development, and administration, with a fair profit margin thrown in.

◆ Government Price Controls

Patent law and health insurance systems in the US versus other countries aren't necessarily all that different. The difference lies in regulations. With apologies to Mr. McKinnell, government price controls, overseen by various government agencies, have put caps on drug prices in other countries. It's this difference, more than anything else, that is the main reason why drugs remain relatively affordable in other industrial nations while being out of control in the United States.

The following chart outlines agencies used by other countries to deal with drug prices:

TABLE 3-1
Approaches to Drug Pricing in Other Countries

	Australia	Canada		Germany	India	United Kingdom
National Organization	Pharmaceutical Benefits Advisory Committee	Patented Medicine Prices Review Board	Canadian Agency for Drugs and Technologies in Health	Federal Joint Committee or the Institute for Quality and Efficiency in Health Care	National Pharmaceutical Pricing Authority	National Institute for Health and Clinical Excellence
Applicability	Public payers	All payers	Public payers except in Quebec (non-cancer drugs)	All insurers	All payers	National Health Service
Review Criteria	Comparative effectiveness, safety, and cost-effectiveness; projected usage and overall costs to the health care system	Therapeutic innovation; comparative pricing with respect to France, Germany, Italy, Sweden, the United Kingdom, and the United States	Comparative effectiveness, safety, and cost-effectiveness; patient experiences	Comparative benefit	National List of Essential Medicines prepared on the basis of efficacy, safety, cost-effectiveness, and common diseases	Clinical effectiveness and cost-effectiveness
Decision	Coverage (yes, no, limited)	Price reductions or rebates	Coverage	Price setting after first year on the market	Formulary inclusion or exclusion	Coverage
Binding	Yes	Yes	No	Yes	Yes	Yes

SOURCE: Adapted and expanded from Kesselheim et al. 2016.

◆ Does It Work?

How well do these agencies work? A 2019 report issued by House Committee on Ways and Means reported the following:

- Six of the seven noninsulin medications used to treat type 2 diabetes were priced 600 percent to 1,100 percent higher in the United States than abroad.
- Humira, an anti-inflammatory drug, is priced at $2,436.02 per dose in the US (or about 500 percent of the international average). The next highest price for the drug is in Denmark, where it costs $787.10 per dose.
- The average cost of Xeljanz, another arthritis medication in the US, is $68.26, versus $20.71 per dose, the average of other countries.
- The average US list price for multiple sclerosis drugs was $769.92 per dose, compared to $133.99 per dose in other countries.
- The US list price for nine cancer medications ranged from $90.88 to $791.66 per dose, averaging approximately $342.48. The international average of these same drugs was $93.29 per dose.

The next question to ask is if, or whether, the United States is taking heed of what is going on in other countries. The answer here is kind of.

In 2018, the Centers for Medicare & Medicaid Services released an Advance Notice of Proposed Rulemarking that attempted to develop and maintain international models to reduce US drug prices. However, while the ANPRM focused more on how Medicare pays for in-office Part B prescription drugs, the model didn't include drugs that patients pay for at the pharmacy, under Medicare Part D. The Trump administration has taken initial stabs at initiating an ERP system, though the first design hasn't taken into account most ERP recommendations.

The model is geared to change how Medicare pays hospitals and providers (but not pharmaceutical companies) for drugs. However, nothing in the proposal requires drug companies to sell the prescriptions to the middleman at a lower price, meaning a concern that such proposals would do little more than shift costs around. Another problem with this proposal is that it's limited to Part B; most drug costs are incurred in Part D, reducing the IPI's ability to affect the drug pricing system on a larger scale for Medicare beneficiaries, or the overall US public. Still, it could be argued that the ANPRM is a step in the right direction, albeit a very small one.

As much as the Hank McKinnells of the word decry regulation of drug prices, claiming that such a move will stifle research and innovation, they fail to take into account that the current do-nothing policy of the United States means consumers continue to be subject to escalating drug prices. The more the prices increase, the less affordable they become and the more nonadherence increases. The higher the degree of nonadherence, the higher the burden on the overall public health system. There is no excuse for this public health crisis, especially as other countries have managed to put a cap on lower drug prices, without causing undue harm to their populations.

The United States should take a good look at this. It could learn some lessons.

The problem we continually face, however, is that any time a government or agency body attempts to step in to do something about higher pharmaceutical prices (or health care prices, in general), some other entity steps in, accusing the government or agency of exceeding its authority. Such challenges seem to be successful more often than not, which explains why the United States' governmental entities appear to be helpless to do much about the current crisis.

THE PRESIDENT AND PRESIDENT-ELECT

BECAUSE ANYTHING TO DO WITH HEALTH CARE (AND BY extension, health care costs) falls into the lap of the federal government, it stands to reason that the federal government's two branches—the executive and legislative—have a great deal of influence on passing laws and ensuring they are enacted. It should also be observed that, at times, the judicial branch steps in as well. At this time, the Affordable Care Act is once again before the US Supreme Court, brought to it by GOP-dominated states and the Trump administration (Totenberg, 2020). And once again, the argument is focused on whether the government has the right to force anyone to acquire health insurance. Whether the court upholds the ACA this time (as before) is anyone's guess. Repealing the ACA could have catastrophic consequences, but that is beyond the scope of this paper. The Trump administration did manage to take out the ACA's health insurance mandate by adding it to the Tax Cuts and Jobs Act of 2017 legislation. This most recent example of ACA under fire continues to demonstrate that health care overall remains a hot-button issue among legislators.

It also remains a concern of presidents. The first president to campaign for national health insurance legislation was Harry Truman in the late 1940s. It seems as though since that time, even as presidents suggest similar improvements to both health care and pharmaceutical costs, pulling any meaningful legislation through literally requires an act of Congress. Congress isn't always so agreeable, due to reasons already mentioned: lobbyists, organizations, and campaign contributors dislike anything that disrupts the profitable status quo. Still, it's an interesting exercise to determine what President Donald Trump has done in an attempt to curtail rising drug prices. It's also an interesting exercise to take a look at President-Elect Joe Biden's stance on pharmaceutical costs and his plans, if any, to reduce them.

◆ President Donald Trump

President Trump has presented a somewhat interesting dichotomy when it comes to health care. While he repeatedly has tried to overturn the Affordable Care Act (an effort that he began during the early months of his presidency), he also has been outspoken about escalating drug prices. In a limited fashion, he's attempted to do something about it. One of his main efforts has involved introducing, and attempting to implement, a blueprint.

In May 2018, President Trump introduced his American Patients First: The Trump Administration Blueprint to Lower Drug Prices and Reduce Out-of-Pocket Costs (HHS, 2018). The blueprint, or plan, was focused on four areas of pharmaceutical reform: improved competition, better negotiation, incentive for lower list prices, and decrease in out-of-pocket costs (HHS, 2018). In this document, the

Trump administration put the blame for skyrocketing pharmaceutical prices on opaque rebates and discounts that support high list prices, the generational loss of patent exclusivity, taxes created by the Affordable Care Act, expansion of the 340B drug discount program, expansion of international price controls, a lack of negotiating power among government programs, and "changes in insurance benefit design that shifted the burden of rising prices to consumers" (HHS, 2018).

Did the Trump administration reach any of its goals? Before moving forward, it's important to understand that the blueprint wasn't developed and issued to take care of every challenge involving pharmaceuticals and prices. Rather, it was issued in two phases, the first of which was actions that the president could direct the Department of Health and Human Services to take immediately (HHS, 2018). The second phase focused on "actions HHS is actively considering, on which feedback is being solicited" (HHS, 2018). In other words, rather than being considered a mandate, the blueprint actually took the form of suggestions. As of now, there is no way of knowing if those "suggestions" are being considered. However, Trump has taken the following actions in attempts to lower drug prices.

Tearing off the Gag

During October 2018, the Trump administration signed two bills into law, banning "gag order" clauses on contracts between pharmacies and insurance companies and pharmacy benefit managers. Before the Know the Lowest Price Act of 2018 (S. 2553) and the Patient Right to Know Drug Prices Act (S. 2554) were signed into law, pharmacists were forbidden from telling customers when, and where, they could pay the pharmacy's lower cash price instead of the price negotiated by their insurance plans. While pharmacists can now explain cheaper alternatives, they are not under any obligation to do so; the pharmacist can tell patients only if they ask (Konrad, 2019). As such, the onus is on the consumer to ask the pharmacist if paying cash will be less expensive than using insurance. Still, the legislation does begin to nibble away at the price secrecy that continually shrouds this industry.

A Plethora of Executive Orders

Another task that Trump has taken on involved signing a series of executive orders in an attempt to lower drug prices. These have included Lowering Prices for Patients by Eliminating Kickbacks to Middlemen and Increasing Drug Importation to Lower Prices for American Patients, both signed on July 24, 2020 (HHS, 2020). These executive orders sought to do everything from "end a shadowy system of kickbacks by middlemen that lurks behind the high out-of-pocket costs many Americans face at the pharmacy counter" to requiring federally qualified health centers that purchase insulin and epinephrine through the 340B program to pass savings from discounted drug prices to medically underserved patients (HHS, 2020).

As an aside, the 340B Drug Pricing Program is directed by HHS, which allows hospitals and clinics serving high volumes of lower-income patients to purchase discounted outpatient drugs

(Orwig, 2018). The program has been in place since 1992 and as of 2013 was estimated to save provider organizations $3.8 billion. These costs, by the way, are not necessarily passed on to the consumer; the plan is in place to assist providers caring for a population that might not be able to afford drugs.

The program, however, generated controversy when the Centers for Medicare and Medicaid (CMS) finalized a rule to cut Medicare Part B reimbursement for drugs purchased at 340B discounts by 28 percent. Providers didn't like this rule because it meant new coding requirements, not to mention the fact they thought CMS had overstated its statutory authority by reducing Medicare payment rates. That challenge is in the courts at this time.

Back to Trump's executive orders, his recent attempt was signed on Sept. 13, 2020: On Lowering Drug Prices by Putting America First. This latter executive order focused on "most-favored nation price," meaning that the Medicare program shouldn't pay more for Part B or Part D prescription drugs or biological products than the price that a drug manufacturer sells in a member country belonging to the OCED (Trump, 2020).

Finally, and until recently, drug imports from other countries were prohibited, except in certain cases, citing safety concerns (Freed, Neuman, and Cubanski, 2020). This hasn't prevented US citizens from driving over the Canadian or Mexican borders in attempts to obtain less-expensive drugs. It is the mass importation of drugs into the US, from these countries, that is banned.

However, in an effort to lower drug costs for Americans, the Trump administration has been working on pathways to allow importation of drugs from Canada. In late 2019, the Trump administration issued a notice of proposed rulemaking; if that is finalized, it would allow the importation of certain, specific drugs from Canada (HHS, 2019). Additionally, the administration announced new draft guidance, describing procedures that drug manufacturers in the US can follow to help facilitate the importation of prescription drugs, such as FDA-approved drugs, that are manufactured abroad and authorized for sale in any foreign country.

But this could prove to be difficult on a nationwide basis. Noted Axene Health Partners (2018), "It would be difficult for the United States to process its drug purchase through a country one-ninth its size."

The main problem with Trump's executive orders is that they don't have much in the way of "teeth." Rather, they seem to be orders and documents that are being put into place in response to a weary public's consistent request for government to "do something" about the continuing escalating prices.

While federal law does grant the president a great deal of authority through executive action, that authority isn't unlimited (Waldrop and Rapfogel, 2020). For one thing, the president can't implement orders or policies that run up against conflicting laws. For instance, a September 13 executive order directs the HHS secretary to launch a rulemaking to test an international reference pricing model, but until that rulemaking is finalized (which includes time needed for public input), the order is meaningless.

Furthermore, and perhaps just as important, the provision allowing the Medicare program to test different payment approaches is embedded in the Affordable Care Act—and the Trump administration is, as mentioned above, trying to overturn it.

Perhaps understandably, Big Pharma is not in favor of any of this. Stephen Ubl, president and CEO of the Pharmaceutical Researcher and Manufacturers of America, indicated that the "favored nation" system is "an irresponsible and unworkable policy that will give foreign governments a say in how America provides access to treatments and cures for seniors and people struggling with devastating diseases (2010)." Meanwhile, Nicole Longo, who is PhRMA's director of public affairs, added that the orders "would allow US politicians to decide what medicines are worth, based on foreign governments' arbitrary determinations of a medicine's value (2020)." She also complained—getting back to the industry's refrain—that the executive order would interfere with Big Pharma's ability to research and develop new medicines, especially in the face of eliminating COVID-19 (Longo, 2020).

Share the Price Information

At one point, the Trump administration directed HHS to mandate the publication of list prices of drugs within direct-to-consumer television advertising, especially targeting prescription drugs covered by Medicare and Medicaid. The purpose of the rule was to increase transparency, thereby (in theory) keeping drug prices low (Armour, 2019). The Trump administration pointed out that list prices mattered to patients, especially those facing large out-of-pocket costs and high deductibles.

Trump went on record (via Twitter) at one point decrying drug companies' secrecy when it came to their prices. "If drug companies are ashamed of those prices," he tweeted, "lower them!" In other words, the idea behind such transparency is to shame the drug manufacturers, thereby prompting them to lower their prices so they don't get more fingers pointed at them.

Again (and not surprisingly) drugmakers opposed the price mandate, suggesting that the rule would improperly limit free speech. In this case, the drug manufacturers have a point, because forcing them to switch the content of their ads to reflect pricing would constitute a free-speech violation. In addition, Ezekiel Emanuel, chair of the Department of Medical Ethics and Health Policy at the University of Pennsylvania, pointed out, perhaps quite rightly, that simply showing drug prices on TV ads won't work because it lacks any type of enforcement mechanism (Alvaro, Challener, and Branch, 2019). Any enforcement mechanism that might be considered for this could, once again, be considered a violation of free speech, which means Congress would not pass such a requirement.

This also doesn't take into account that showing manufacturers prices on DTC advertising will muddy the waters. At this point, the actual costs of drugs are highly individualized, shaped by everything from PBM influence to pharmacy markups and insurance plan requirements. In other words, a higher price for a pharmaceutical shown in an ad could end up being much lower once the consumer actually acquires it. And showing a high price for a drug could have negative consequences in that it could deter those in need of treatment because they believe they wouldn't be able to afford the drug.

Furthermore, shaming the pharmaceutical companies into lowering their prices on drugs hasn't been effective, and there's no reason why splashing prices on television or in magazines would do anything more. Said Emanuel,

> Part of the Trump administration's theory seems to be that by shaming drug companies, they might lower their prices. But nothing seems to shame them. Indeed, after all the uproar over $600 EpiPens, EpiPens are, well, still $600. (Alvaro, Challener, and Branch, 2019)

It should come as no surprise that a lawsuit was brought against this rule by Merck, Eli Lilly, and Amgen Inc. (Armour, 2019). And it should also be no surprise that a federal judge ultimately blocked the "show-me-the-price" rule in July 2019. According to US District Judge Amit Mehta in Washington DC, the HHS rules would violate free speech while exceeding the agency's statutory authority. As misguided as this thought was, it does provide a good example of both the power of the pharmaceutical industry and constant challenges to agency oversight.

With all of the above, the logical issue is whether Trump's blueprint has been at all effective. Certainly, legislation getting rid of the pharmacist gag order is one small step in the right direction. And overall, Trump's blueprint has been well-meaning, whether it's ascribed to political rhetoric or the president sincerely wanted to see a decline in high prescription costs. The problem, however, was that it lacked specific proposals that could be put into action, nor did it target the actual problem inherent in all of this, which are the price mechanisms when it comes to prescription drugs. Furthermore, because the proposals do require regulatory reaction (spearheaded by the Department of Health and Human Services), immediate action isn't anticipated.

Washington, DC, reporter Stephen Barlas (2018) pointed out that "the fact that drug companies are sitting on the edge of their seats waiting for the administration to put a plan into place doesn't mean a plan will evolve quickly. It clearly won't" (p. 606). Six weeks after the blueprint was released, Health and Human Services Secretary Alex Azur told the Senate Health, Education, Labor, and Pensions Committee that his department certainly has the authority to force drug companies to disclose their list prices in television advertisements. The problem, however, is that without legislation backing that authority, pharmaceutical manufacturers could challenge it in court (Barlas, 2018) as indeed they have.

Azur also told the committee that he would like to see legislation eliminating the 100 percent cap on drug rebates imposed by the ACA, creating an incentive for drug companies to raise list prices (Barlas, 2018). Again, though, Congress isn't exactly racing to do any of this.

Finally, the stakeholders involved have disagreed on this plan. Barlas noted that the 3,000 comments on the blueprint initially show support of the Trump administration's efforts to lower drug prices. "Then they all degenerate into opposition to most of the Blueprint's suggestions," Barlas wrote (p. 608).

This leads to the crux of the matter. Presidents can say what they want about health care reform—whether it involves nationalizing the health care system or bringing down prescription costs. But without legislation to actively back any of it, pharmaceutical companies will be more than happy to bring rulings, rulemaking, and executive orders to the courts to determine their constitutionality. The problem here is that lowering drug prices is a marathon, not a quick win. That marathon has a lot of racers, not all of whom have the consumers' best interests in mind.

◆ President-Elect Joe Biden

The question then needs to be asked, "Can the president-elect do better?" Unlike Trump, Biden has had experience in dealing with the harsh political realities of any kind of health care reform. He was, after all, vice president when President Barack Obama signed the Patient Protection and Affordable Care Act of 2010. Biden understood the hoops the Obama administration had to go through to get that piece of legislation through (not to mention the repeated challenges for repeal it continues to undergo). He understood the myriad agencies, constituents, and others involved with the entire process. People might not remember now, but getting the ACA through Congress required a great deal of negotiation, not to mention appeals to public reason. Once again, any kind of meaningful reform requires a lot of effort and resources directed toward the issue.

However, we know that Biden has some thoughts about pharmaceutical reform, based on some of his campaign comments. For instance, Biden indicated that he plans to eliminate the barrier preventing Medicare from using its leveraging power to negotiate drug prices (Archer, 2020). He also proposes the formation of a new arm of Health and Human Services to assess the value of new specialty drugs; the agency would establish a fair price on such drugs, basing it on international pricing if the drug is already available in other countries (Archer, 2020). Other proposals the president-elect put forward include the following:

- imposing a limit on the amount pharmaceutical companies can increase the prices of their brand-name and biotech drugs, pinning that increase to the rate of inflation. The limit would also apply to "abusively priced" generics (though the president-elect never really defines what this means)
- allowing drug importation from other countries in which the drugs are deemed to be safe
- allowing private health insurers in the state exchanges to benefit from HHS-established prescription drug prices
- eliminating tax deductions pharmaceutical companies current receive on advertising spending
- improving the supply of generic drugs

One cause for concern about drug pricing under a Biden presidency is that the pharmaceuticals and health products industry donated more than $5.9 million to his presidential campaign, versus less than $1.5 million going to Trump (Roche, 2020). This has led experts and industry stakeholders to wonder if this might color Biden's ability to introduce a comprehensive plan to lower costs. It could be assumed that he is in the pocket with Big Pharma. But others wonder if the accelerated donations were in place to "keep him and Congress from turning his drug-pricing proposals into law" (Archer, 2020).

At this time, it's way too soon to tell if—or whether—Biden will focus his attention on pharmaceutical costs. His first order of business when finally sworn in will be handling the spread of COVID-19. However, if he is able to undo the ban on Medicare negotiation processes, that would be another small step in the right direction.

SOLUTIONS

AS I'VE SHOWN THROUGHOUT THIS BOOK, HIGH PRE-
scription prices are not the purview of just one entity. As easy as it
might be to blame the pharmaceutical manufacturers, they are only
one part of the problem. Reforms along the entire pharmaceutical
change would be necessary in an effort to lower prices in a meaningful fashion.

Many good ideas have been introduced in an attempt to lower
prices. These include transparency of pricing, with public disclo-
sure at each step of the drug supply chain (Mathew, Kilpatrick, and
Garber, 2019). State boards of experts should also be formed to
examine prescription drug pricing, based on transparency. Other
solutions have also been offered. Patent reform legislation, reference
pricing, outcome-based pricing, and providing incentives to physicians and pharmacists to prescribe lower-price drugs have been
some of the solutions introduced to bring down higher drug prices
(van der Gronde, Uyl-de Groot, and Pieters, 2017).

The main problem with many drug reform ideas, however, is that
they don't have a holistic intent. Rather, they are put forth to change

one part of the system. The Medicare legislation, for example, provides information about what is covered and how much beneficiaries can save but does nothing to exert price controls over the pharmaceutical supply chain. (Such controls would be "un-American," at least, from the point of view of those within the industry.)

Furthermore, before any kind of pricing reform is pushed through, Khullar and Bach (2020) point out that, first and foremost, it's important to realize that drugs undergo a three-stage period or journey.

1) Innovation. The innovation period is when new products are tested, developed, and prepared to be submitted to the FDA.

2) Monopoly. If the drugs are approved (most are not), the next step is the monopoly period, during which they are protected from competition by the FDA exclusivities and through patents.

3) Competitive. Once the patents expire and exclusivity period ends, other companies can manufacturer and sell the brand-name drug, either under another brand name or as a generic.

The authors point out that adjusting incentives along any part of this "journey" could potentially help with pricing. The authors also offer the following suggestions:

1) Link innovation-friendly policies to price concessions. The idea here is that there are ways to reduce risks of failure and costs of innovation to drug companies, which don't rely on those companies charging exorbitant prices. In recent periods,

regulations have been introduced to push drugs more quickly through the review process, which can save companies hundreds of millions of dollars, savings that are hoped would be passed on to consumers. Back in 1981, Congress created tax credits to offset research costs, while Medicare began covering medical expenses for patients in clinical trials, beginning in 2000. The innovation-friendly policies haven't been linked to price concessions from drug companies in the past but should be considered for the future.

2) Revamp how long new drugs can enjoy monopoly protection. To reiterate, the FDA typically gives companies five to twelve years of exclusive rights to sell a new drug after approval, while patent protections can last for decades. This is because manufacturers often patent not just original molecules, but also minor changes to the drug, such as its coating, shape, or even how it can be administered. In one example, the biologic Enbrel, which has been on the market since the 1990s to treat inflammatory conditions such as rheumatoid arthritis, is well beyond the FDA's exclusivity protection. However, its mass of patents—running more than one hundred deep—don't expire until 2029, with the drug currently costing nearly $70,000 per year. In these cases, the bullet needs to be bitten, with the number and types of patents available to drug manufacturers reduced. This would help limit how long patients and taxpayers are exposed to higher prices.

3) Remove all obstacles to competition from generics. Policymakers have been notoriously slow when it comes

to removing barriers that generic drug manufacturers face when trying to enter the market. The above-mentioned "pay-for-delay" tactic is one such way in which generic competition has been removed, with little done to correct it. Drug companies also use other tools to prevent competition before it begins. For instance, drug companies will cite safety concerns in refusing to provide samples that generic manufacturers need to prove that their products are equivalent to branded drugs. The Creating and Restoring Equal Access to Equivalent Samples Act of 2019 (CREATES), was signed into law in December 2019 to target delay tactics used to block development of affordable, FDA-approved generic and biosimilar medicines. Still, evergreening, product hopping, and pay-for-delay still exist.

The Federal Trade Commission could help here by stepping in and more aggressively enforcing antitrust laws against these tactics. The FTC should also keep a better eye on pharmacy benefit managers' "rebating" practices. Such a practice is not "discounting" but a kickback. Meanwhile, the FDA could do more, such as not granting market exclusivity, based only on pharmaceuticals that been cosmetically changed, especially right before branded products are set to lose monopoly protections. Specifically, both the FDA and FTC need to do a much better job of using current laws to force pharmaceutical companies and pharmaceutical benefit managers into better behavior. Perhaps this will also end the finger-pointing for higher prices between these two entities.

However, the above proposals—or any other health care-oriented proposal for that matter—won't go anywhere without the backing or support of Congress, which continues to be a constant bottleneck in this situation. Added to the mix is that "the biopharmaceutical sector is fraught with discordant viewpoints, divergent priorities, and conflicts of interest that can impede the provision of quality health care, especially to socioeconomically disadvantaged populations" (Augustine, Madhavan, and Nass, 2018, p. 3).

This is another crux of the matter. Let's get back to President Trump's executive orders. Even assuming that these orders did have "teeth" and could be immediately enacted upon, they wouldn't delve into the fact that the pharmaceutical industry is a highly fragmented one.

Furthermore, such a solution assumes that Big Pharma will do nothing about more drugs coming to the US from Canada. This is patently not the case. (Let's not forget that the pharmaceutical industry has no problem challenging presidential executive orders in court.) The industry's likely response to such a move would be for drug manufacturers to limit drug production and sales to Canada, in an effort to increase prices there (Axene Health Partners, 2018). This would hurt Canadian consumers while potentially leading to passage of laws prohibiting the exportation of drugs to the United States. In other words, allowing importation of drugs without taking into account the entire big picture of the industry would lead to a larger mess than the one we are currently facing.

Additionally, allowing drug imports from Canada or comparing US drug prices to other "favored nations" tackles one arm of this confusing octopus. What it doesn't do, however, is take pharmacy benefit managers and their opaque pricing and rebates out of the equation.

It's no wonder that Ann Marie Marciarille (2017), professor of law at the University of Missouri at Kansas City, agreed, pointing out that "different solutions are likely appropriate for different problems in different segments of the pharmaceutical market" (p. 46).

Marciarille also indicated that the current pharmaceutical pricing challenge—involving questions concerning access and affordability—is also a public health challenge. One problem is that finding a one-size-fits-all solution can be highly difficult as "we consume pharmaceutical drugs individually according to our unique profiles," meaning that "we experience problems of cost and access individually" (Marciarille, 2017, p. 45). Furthermore, another issue is that the fair competition/antitrust laws and public health laws aren't on the same page when it comes to pharmaceuticals. "The former cannot agree on the relevant definition of consumer welfare. The latter does not fully comprehend the highly complex, but inherently collective nature of pharmaceutical drug acquisition in the United States," according to Marciarille (p. 45).

Because of this, controlling high prices rests with more than one stakeholder. For instance, private health insurance companies should modify their plans in order to reduce financial burdens that might be incurred by patients and their families, if costly prescription drugs are needed for treatment. Along those lines, individual cost-sharing arrangements based on drug prices should be calculated as a fraction of the net purchase price rather than manufacturers' list prices. Furthermore, PBMs could steer utilization toward more cost-effective drugs, rather than putting forward the pricier versions.

PBMs should also change the ways in which they are paid.

Doing this would remove incentives that make already high drug prices even higher (Gill, 2020). The Pharmaceutical Research and Manufacturers of America backs this plan; the organization, in fact, suggests that PBMs receive a flat fee for the work they do rather than a negotiated rebate payment. Moving down this path would help lead to transparent pricing, while reducing many of the administrative costs that tend to lead to higher pricing.

In all fairness, private insurers have started sharing drug rebates with their members, which is one step in the right direction. But again, given the many stakeholders involved with drug pricing, the main solutions will likely rest in the hands of government, physicians, and even consumers. What follows are some suggestions that could help.

◆ What the Government Can Do

Frankly, the government needs to do a better job of stepping in and controlling drug prices. Federal entities, especially, need to evade charges of "socialism" whenever they try to pass something through that might rein in skyrocketing costs. Let's face it: Big Pharma, pharmacy benefit managers, and insurance companies aren't going to do a thing about it; this industry has spectacularly failed at any kind of reasonable pricing activities. This industry has been consistently shamed by the media and public, put under a congressional microscope, and lambasted by consumers and health care trade organizations, such as the American Medical Association and American Hospital Association. But things continue as they are.

What needs to be emphasized, realized, and understood is that the industry's claims it is operating on a free-market system are simply not true. The sooner everyone realizes this, the less afraid (hopefully) government will be when it comes to stepping in and taking control. A free-market system implies that, first and foremost, consumers can make a rational choice when it comes to purchasing a good or service. In truth, consumers don't make a decision as to whether or not to buy a particular drug. Rather, their health care providers make those decisions. The insurance companies also make the decisions as to whether a drug can be covered. This means consumers are, in a sense, buying a product decided on by other entities.

Second, a free-market system operates by supply and demand. Specifically, manufacturers supply a good or service based on demand for that service. With pharmaceuticals, however, it doesn't seem as though this is happening. Rather than supplying an actual drug to meet an actual need (such as better treatments for glioblastoma multiforme), the industry continues to put money-makers into the system. Certainly high cholesterol, high blood pressure, congestive heart failure, and even erectile dysfunction require treatment. But rather than gauging the demand for such drugs, pharmaceutical manufacturers simply add to already existing products. Adding insult to this injury, the FDA is doing nothing to stem this tide.

Finally, this is an industry that enjoys unprecedented pricing power and gets away with it. This is due to patent protections and market exclusivities. Certainly, drug companies need a way to recoup their expenses. No one is denying that these companies deserve a profit either. However, they also should not be permitted to go out of their way to take advantage of loopholes in the system, which is happening. In any other industry, the Federal Trade Commission and other agencies would come down harshly on pharma's stakeholders with claims of everything from collusion to restriction of competition. Yet for whatever the reason, government agencies and Congress have taken a hands-off attitude toward the pharmaceutical industry, most likely out of fear.

This needs to stop. One major step the government can—and must—take is to consolidate and apply purchasing power directly to negotiate prices with producers and suppliers of medicines, while strengthening formulary design and management.

As I pointed out above, other industrialized, Western nations have a specific, central negotiating agency to ensure negotiating power. The largest difference between US drug prices and those within other developed nations is that those nations have a board or committee that is responsible for negotiating directly with drug companies, thereby bringing down prices. This is in direct opposition to what we, in the United States, face, which is a patchwork quilt of federal and state regulations. This has led to vast differences in drug prices, not just by state but by municipality and even pharmacy.

Federal entities must be encouraged to negotiate drug prices, including on behalf of state agencies that might want to be represented. This means, for example, that the Medicare Modernization Act must be amended to give Medicare negotiating power.

It should come as no surprise that drug companies argue that such a centralized negotiation policy could limit access to treatment and therapies. This complaint is nonsense. Between 2013 and 2017, the five largest US-based drug companies spent 70 percent more on marketing and administrative costs than on research and development (House Committee on Ways and Means, 2019). Furthermore, from 2006 to 2015, the twenty-five largest pharmaceutical companies' average sales revenues increased by $241 billion, while funding they dedicated to research and development increased only by $7 billion. As such, the supposed high costs of research and development seem to be only a small fraction of what Big Pharma actually earns on a yearly basis.

Centralizing negotiations and decreasing fragmentation is one step the government can take to help with costs.

In its report "Making Medicines Affordable: A National Imperative," the National Academies of Sciences, Engineering, and Medicine suggests that the government should also consider the following in reducing out-of-control prescription drug prices:

1) Accelerate market entry, and use, of safe and effective generics. Along these lines, it means the government should step in and foster competition in an effort to boost affordability and availability of products. To do this, agencies such as the FTC need to crack down on shady practices by pharmaceutical manufacturers, such as product-hopping, evergreening, and pay-to-delay.

2) Eliminate patent loopholes. The FDA needs to step in and stop pharma manufacturers from issuing new patents on already existing drugs simply because they want to change a pill's color. This is not a "new" drug. It is a change to an old one. New patents on existing drugs can be applied for if the drug will be undergoing a major change. Otherwise,

patents should be allowed to expire and competition should be allowed in.

3) Require greater price transparency along the pharmaceutical supply chain. While this is one aspect issued by Trump's blueprint, it didn't go far enough. The blueprint requirement focused only on direct-to-consumer advertising, which is not the place to be revealing how much a drug costs.

In reality, pricing of drugs is very convoluted and opaque. Pharmaceutical "list prices" are secret. PBM rebates are secret. Until recently, pharmacists couldn't even tell consumers which drug was more expensive than another. The secrecy needs to stop, with all pharmaceutical stakeholders required to disclose prices paid, including net prices received and paid, discounts, and rebates. This information could be published in a National Drug Code issued on a quarterly basis. Along these lines, pharmaceutical companies should be required to submit an annual public report stating list prices, rebates, and discounts to payers. This would be far better than revealing prices on a late-night television ad.

4) Discourage direct-to-consumer advertising of prescription drugs and direct financial incentives for patients. One issue that has been consistently brought up in this paper is that direct-to-consumer advertising puts awareness of more expensive drugs in the minds of patients, thus creating a demand for the drug versus its lower-cost counterpart. We need to make one thing clear, however: direct-to-consumer advertising has always been around. One only needs to take a look at the snake-oil advertisements from the late nineteenth

and early twentieth centuries to see this. But for the most part, the pharmaceutical industry was fairly circumspect about advertising their drugs. In fact, at one point, the industry was reluctant to embark on direct-to-consumer activities, believing that doing so would hurt the doctor-patient relationship and confused a public that knew little about drugs or had little understanding of risk/reward or cost/benefits of the drugs.

However, the combination of increased consumerism in health care, and the FDA's relaxation of rules about what pharmaceutical manufacturers could promote in their products, seemed to open the floodgates for today's ads.

One way in which the government can reduce DTC advertising is to eliminate the tax deductibility of those advertising expenses. Furthermore, patient coupon programs should be eliminated, except in cases in which there is no competing drug in the marketplace.

This is not to suggest, however, that communication or information should be totally cut off from consumers. Patients are certainly entitled to obtain information about particular drugs. It would be far better for the government to encourage pharmaceutical companies to provide specific, useful efficacy information to patients. Such information could include benefits of treatment, potential costs, and options. The FDA should also re-implement the requirement that side effects need to be listed. Moving away from glitzy advertising into better information could go a long way toward reducing demand for the higher-priced drugs.

Finally, the government needs to reduce the scope and length of monopolies. The patents are understandable—the exclusivity periods, not so much. A drug that provides little or no incremental value over existing products receives the same patent/exclusivity protections and ability to charge monopolistic prices for an extended period of time (Engelberg, 2015). Basically, a tweak to a drug that has been on the market for more than twenty years receives the same protection as a new, blockbuster drug that can delay cancerous growth. The current system of exclusivities needs to be scrapped and replaced by a system that rewards research-producing drugs of high therapeutic value, which can be a benefit to society.

The above suggestions will require agencies and Congress to ignore the criticisms of pharmaceutical manufacturers and focus on what will be best for the US consumer. There is absolutely no reason why consumers shouldn't have access to safe, affordable generics. There is also no reason why consumers should be consistently bombarded by a host of prescription advertisements.

◆ What Physicians/Prescribers Can Do

Having indicated above what government should do, the reality is it likely won't happen any time soon. As much as we hope it will happen, the FDA won't suddenly put rules into place overthrowing patents or exclusivity. Nor will Congress pass any kind of law that restricts prices increases of drugs. Again, getting meaningful health care reform pushed into law a decade ago created a huge uproar. It's not likely that this will be tried again anytime soon. While insurance companies and PBMs can do their part (see the above suggestions), it's also up to the end users—physicians and consumers—to focus on ways to cut costs.

Physicians are the first step in helping curtail prices, which can be done through the following suggestions (Fiscella, Venci, Sanders, Lanigan, and Fortunua, 2019):

1) Encourage staff to screen patients in terms of medication costs.

    When a patient and intake nurse first sit down, the nurse proceeds to ask a variety of questions, ranging from physical complaints to prescribed medications. What does not seem to be asked, however, is if the patient has the financial means to afford those medications. As such, one of the questions that should be asked of patients during the intake activities should involve any financial burdens a patient might face when it comes to medications. One problem that can be faced by health care providers is that patients won't automatically volunteer the fact that they might not be able to afford medication, either because of pride or because they think no affordable options are available. This can lead to nonadherence. On the plus side, patients are more likely to share information about cost concerns and nonadherent behavior with nursing or other office staff as opposed to talking with their physicians. As such, asking the question about a patient's finances, in a tactful way, can help determine whether that patient can afford drugs.

2) Focus on brief, cost-reduction strategies during visits.

    Again, this goes under the assumption that a patient won't willingly tell a doctor that he or she can't afford a particular drug that is prescribed. Instead, it's up to the doctor or health care provider to confirm any cost concerns, such as discussing unmet deductibles or out-of-pocket costs, that might come with prescribing the particular drug. With this information in hand, the health care provider can come up with more cost-effective solutions to assist the patient and to ensure compliance. Such solutions can include issuing free samples or prescribing less-costly but just as effective medications.

Physicians and other health care providers should also educate themselves about various apps and tools that can be used to help decrease the costs of drugs. For instance, apps such as www.goodrx.com provide comparative costs between pharmacies as well as offer coupons for prescription medications. Others along these same lines include SingleCare, WellRx, and RxSaver.

3) When necessary, refer patients who need more assistance to other services.

Navigating insurance plans can be difficult as can determining eligibility for additional insurance coverage, such as low-income subsidies or applying for pharmaceutical medication assistance programs. Referring to case/care managers or social workers can be helpful in such situations. If these resources aren't available, another member of the staff should be assigned to provide assistance and to champion the efforts made to focus on reducing costs.

In addition to solutions proposed by Fiscella et al., another way in which health care providers can help reduce costs is to tap into reference-pricing programs. These identify a reference drug in each category, which is the lowest-cost clinical equivalent to one or more higher-priced drugs (Henka, 2018). This in turn could mean lower prices are available to consumers for a drug that has a similar therapeutic use to its higher-priced counterpart. This solution could also give the consumer the choice. If he or she doesn't want the lower-price drug, reference pricing allows him or her to pay the difference in cost between the reference drug and the brand-name drug (Henka, 2018). As an aside, in answering the question as to why a patient might not want to pay a low price, some patients are naturally skeptical of generics and lower-priced drugs. This solution gives them a way in which they can still receive some reimbursement for a particular drug, while providing piece-of-mind.

4) Stop giving in to pharma representatives.

While it's tempting to have a pharmaceutical company pay for continuing education courses (or even to provide tickets to some sporting event or concert), physicians need to resist this temptation. The pharmaceutical representatives will do what they can to encourage physicians to prescribe their drugs to patients, even with less costly products available. Physicians also need to stop being speaking shills for pharmaceutical companies. Again, while there is nothing inherently illegal when it comes to taking money from a drug company to speak in support of a particular drug, it does bring up ethical issues. Again, speaking on behalf of a particular drug guarantees that this drug will be prescribed in higher dosages, even if less-costly alternatives are available.

5) Stop automatically reaching for the prescription pad.

Finally, physicians should stop automatically reaching for the prescription pad when it comes to dealing with disease. We've seen what happens when prescriptions are overprescribed and overused. The results can range from antibiotic resistance to opioid addictions. As such, physicians should have a better focus on evidence-based practice when it comes to drugs rather than taking the easy way out. Certainly, this type of thing takes more time to research. But this is the job of the physician.

Overall, the Hippocratic ideal of "first, do no harm" involves more than making patients feel better. This also should include intelligent, thoughtful responses to providing proper cures. This also includes doing no harm to a patient's wallet. Whenever possible, a physician's prescribing habits should focus on the best treatment option that a patient is able to afford.

◆ What Consumers Can Do

We are living in a time of unprecedented consumerism when it comes to health care. Thanks to the internet, anyone can log on to Mayo Clinic or WebMD to research any symptom or potential illness as well as to determine any treatment for that potential illness. Furthermore, consumers are regularly exposed to DTC drug advertising, which provides an overview of what drugs are available to handle various diseases or problems.

Given that consumers are becoming masters of their own

destinies as it pertains to diagnoses and researching disease and illness, consumers should also take extra time to focus on ensuring they aren't on the hook for higher drug costs. This means consumers must stop assuming that everything the pharma industry and health care providers tell them are absolutes and must start being their own advocates, especially when it comes to the potential of utilizing less-expensive drugs.

Consumers are also not well-served by a pharmaceutical industry that continues its advertising bombardment. Big Pharma dedicates an average of 30 percent of its revenues to marketing and creating awareness for specific drug brands (Henka, 2018). Furthermore, they will invest most heavily in their higher-margin drugs (Henka, 2018).

As such, consumers should do the following to ensure they receive the right medications, while reducing expenses:

1) Ask for generics, when possible. Many consumers assume that prescribers will automatically prescribe generics. This is not always the case. There is absolutely nothing wrong in asking a doctor or other health care provider for a generic substitution. And if the answer is no, consumers have every right to ask why.

   Along these lines, consumers should refrain from being "brand snobs" when it comes to medication. Many times, consumers will opt for the higher-price, branded drug, believing that if something costs more, it's better (Henka, 2018). When it comes to pharmaceutical pricing and promotion, this perception has been reinforced. One 2015 study demonstrated that 26 percent of consumers are willing to pay a premium (often as much as 300 percent) for a brand-name headache remedy when an identical store brand is placed right next to it on the shelf. Yet when it comes to comparing the store brand with the nationally branded remedy, the ingredients stack up as exactly the same. The same holds true for pharmaceuticals. Duloxetine provides the same ingredients to help patients with depression and pain as its brand-name counterpart, Cymbalta. As such, consumers should demand the generic drug to save on copays and out-of-pocket costs.

A more specific example involves the brand-name drug Lipitor, which is prescribed for high cholesterol. Lipitor has an average cost of $184 while atorvastatin, the generic version containing the same active ingredient as Lipitor, costs just $36. Meanwhile, simvastatin, a therapeutic drug equivalent, which has a different active ingredient but the same impact on the treatment of the underlying disease, costs just $7. This means that insurance plans with a top-tier copay of $40 for Lipitor are spending $108 more per dose, versus a $0 copay for the generic, and $137 more per dose than the clinical equivalent. If this is the case, why aren't more patients placed on simvastatin? One reason is resistance by PBMs in undermining the payment structures they already have in place with manufacturer partners. Another is, once again, patient perception. The belief is that the Lipitor brand is automatically superior to its generic counterpart or less-expensive equivalent. This is not at all the case. Consumers need to move away from the "more-expensive-is-better" mindset of drugs and focus on the cost-savings of generics that provide the same efficacy and relief of symptoms.

2) Share cost concerns with both physicians and pharmacists. Another way in which consumers can be caught with having to pay higher prices for drugs is that they don't mention the fact they are on fixed incomes, might not have the right insurance, or simply can't afford the higher-priced drug. If consumers are honest and upfront with their health care providers, those providers will work to find more cost-effective medication equivalents.

3) Compare prices between different pharmacies. Most consumers will perform price comparisons on everything from boxed macaroni to chairs. Yet when it comes to pharmaceuticals, they are reluctant to compare prices between pharmacies. One reason for this is because setting up an account at a new pharmacy for prescriptions is inconvenient. However, in the world we currently live in, a little inconvenience is necessary to save money on drugs. Furthermore, apps such as GoodRx can help provide an honest view of what pharmacies will charge, depending on what PBM contract is has negotiated for which drug.

   Taking this one step further, consumers should also be aware of what "tier" a drug might be on a particular insurance plan. If a less-expensive but equally effective drug can be swapped out, it should be considered.

4) Consider using cash rather than insurance. There are times in which paying cash could be less expensive than filing an insurance claim for a pharmaceutical (Konrad, 2019). This is because a retail pharmacy might offer discounts on a drug,

which would make paying cash less expensive than the co-pay that insurance companies or PBMs have negotiated for the same drug (Konrad, 2019). Adding to this, the two laws passed in October 2018 mean pharmacists are required to let consumers know if a cash price for a pharmaceutical is less than an insurance price. However, the consumer must ask, as the pharmacist is not obligated to share that information. It's possible that, if asked, pharmacists can often find discounts or in-store details for a particular drug (Gill, 2020). Returning to the Lipitor example, this typically comes with a $40 copay under many insurance plans (Konrad, 2019). But pharmacies offering a discount might charge only $9 for the full cash price.

Above all, consumers need to rid themselves of the perception that providers and pharmacists will automatically have the best interests, pricewise, of the consumer in mind. This is not always the case. None of this should imply that pharmacists or doctors are shady, dishonest, or simply greedy. But consumers need to not be satisfied with the status quo, especially if that status quo ends up being pricey. While it is the doctor who prescribes a particular medication and the pharmacist who distributes it, it's up to the consumer to find out the best treatment at the best cost and to target the best distribution point from which he or she can buy the medicine on a cost-effective basis.

CONCLUSION: A LONG WAY TO GO

THERE IS ABSOLUTELY NO DOUBT THAT COSTS FOR PHAR-
maceuticals in the United States continue to skyrocket. Government
agencies acknowledge it, health care providers acknowledge it, government and private insurance companies acknowledge it, and consumers are bearing the brunt of it. Even the pharmaceutical manufacturers themselves acknowledge it; neither Mylan's Brescher nor
Norstrum's Mulye denied charging high prices for their respective
drugs. Furthermore, the latter believes it's OK to do so, that drug
companies absolutely have the right to charge as much as the market
will bear.

And if the health care market were similar to a market for ap-
pliances, involving supply and demand and pricing based on these,
Mulye would be absolutely correct. But the health care market in
general and the pharmaceutical market specifically don't operate on
laws of supply and demand, simply because it is so costly to research
and develop a drug and to bring it to market. This is why drugmakers
don't make drugs based on demand. Rather, they make drugs based
on what will make the most money, then they'll create demand by
targeting physicians and consumers through various methods. The

US government is complicit in this effort by encouraging monopolistic practices and pricing, which simply adds to the problem. And whether it's from fear, lobbyists, or campaign contributions (or all of the above), Congress isn't going to do much to rein in these costs.

The problem is that something needs to be done, and done sooner rather than later. The current situation shuts people out from affordable care, and it is unsustainable. It could also lead to a public health crisis from which the nation would be hard-pressed to recover. Certainly, patients and their health care providers can take steps to help reduce costs. But wholesale change is necessary for the industry—change that would include better transparency, less fragmentation, higher negotiating power, and an elimination of patent and monopoly loopholes.

All stakeholders involved with this industry need to take responsibility for reining in costs rather than nibbling at the problem in a piecemeal fashion. Only when these are deployed will we see meaningful change in the area of pharmaceutical pricing.

REFERENCES

American College of Allergy, Asthma & Immunology (ACAAI). 2014. *Epinephrine Auto-Injector.* https://acaai.org/allergies/allergy-treatment/epinephrine-auto-injector.

Aitken, M., E. R. Berndt, and D. M. Cutler. 2008. "Prescription Drug Spending Trends in the United States: Looking beyond the Turning Point." *Health Affairs* 27 no. S1 (December): 151–60. doi:10.1377/hlthaff.28.1.w151.

Alghanem, N., M. Abokwidir, A. B. Fleischer, S. R. Feldman, and W. Alghanem. 2017. "Variation in Cash Price of the Generic Medications Most Prescribed by Dermatologists in Pharmacies across the United States." *Journal of Dermatological Treatment* 28 (2): 119–28. doi:10.1080/09546634.2016.1182614.

Alpert, A., D. Lakdawalla, and N. Snood. 2015. *Prescription Drug Advertising and Drug Utilization: The Role of Medicare Part D.* National Bureau of Economic Research (NBER). https://www.nber.org/system/files/working_papers/w21714/w21714.pdf.

Alvaro, D., Challener, C. A., and Branch, E. (2019, March 12). *Balancing Ethical and Fiduciary Responsibilities in Drug Pricing.* Retrieved from Pharma's Almanac: https://www.

pharmasalmanac.com/articles/balancing-ethical-and-fiduciar
y-responsibilities-in-drug-pricing.

American Academy of Actuaries. (2018, March). *Prescription Drug Spending in the US Healthcare System.* Retrieved from American Academy of Actuaries: https://www.actuary.org/content/ prescription-drug-spending-us-health-care-system.

Andrews, M. (2019, March 29). *The Doughnut Hole Is Gone, but Medicare's Uncapped Drug Costs Still Bite into Budgets.* Retrieved from KHN: https://khn.org/news/doughnut-hole-is-gone-bu t-medicares-uncapped-drug-costs-still-bite-into-budgets/.

Archer, D. (2020, October 14). *What Would a President Biden Do about Drug Prices?* Retrieved from JustCare: https://justcareusa. org/what-would-a-president-biden-do-about-drug-prices/.

Armour, S. (2019, July 8). "Trump Rule Requiring Drug Prices in TV Ads Blocked." Retrieved from *Wall Street Journal:* https:// www.wsj.com/articles/trump-rule-requiring-drug-prices-in -tv-ads-blocked-11562634281.

Augustine, N. R., Madhavan, G., and Nass, S. J., Eds. (2018). *Making Medicines Affordable: A National Imperative.* Washington, DC: National Academies of Sciences, Engineering, and Medicine.

Axene Health Partners. (2018). *US Pharmaceutical Pricing: An Overview.* Retrieved from Axene Health Partners: https:// axenehp.com/us-pharmaceutical-pricing-overview/.

Baker, D. (2006, January). *The Savings from an Efficient Medicare Prescription Drug Plan.* Retrieved from Denter for Economic and Policy Research: https://www.cepr.net/documents/efficient_ medicare_2006_01.pdf.

Barrueta, T. (2015, May 15). *A Brief History of Drug Pricing.* Retrieved from Alliance of Community Health Plans: https://achp.org/wp-content/uploads/Tony-Barrueta-Presentation-5_15_15.pdf.

Barlas, S. (2018, October). Views Conflict on Trump's Drug-Pricing Blueprint. *Pharmacy & Therapeutics, 43*(10), 606–608.

Beaubien, J. (2012, October 15). *Wiping Out Polio: How the US Snuffed Out a Killer.* Retrieved from NPR's *All Things Considered:* https://www.npr.org/sections/health-shots/2012/10/16/162670836/wiping-out-polio-how-the-u-s-snuffed-out-a-killer.

Bennett, C. (2020, April 20). *History of Thalidomide.* Retrieved from News-Medical Net: https://www.news-medical.net/health/History-of-Thalidomide.aspx.

Bluth, R. (2019, April 9). *Can Someone Tell Me What a PBM Does?* Retrieved from KHN: https://khn.org/news/senate-hearing-drug-pricing-lesson-on-pharmacy-benefit-managers/.

Boomershine, C. S. (2010). "Pregabalin for the Management of Fibromyalgia Syndrome." *Journal of Pain Research, 3,* 81–88. doi:10.2147/jpr.s7884.

Briesacher, B., Ross-Degnan, D., Adams, A., Wagner, A., Gurwitz, J., and Soumerai, S. (2009, November-December). "A New Measure of Medication Affordability." *Social Work in Public Health,* 600–612. doi:10.1080/19371910802672346.

Brody, J. E. (2017, April 17). *The Cost of Not Taking Your Medicine.* Retrieved from *New York Times:* https://www.nytimes.com/2017/04/17/well/the-cost-of-not-taking-your-medicine.html.

Caffrey, M. (2018, June 18). *"UpWell Health Survey: 45% of Those with Diabetes Skip Care Due to Costs."* Retrieved from *American Journal of Managed Care:* https://www.ajmc.com/view/upwell-healt h-survey-45-of-those-with-diabetes-skip-care-due-to-costs.

Campbell, T. (2019, May 31). *Is the $2.1 Million Price Tag for Novartis' Zolgensma Ridiculous?* Retrieved from The Motley Fool: https://www.fool.com/investing/2019/05/31/industr y-focus-healthcare-05-29-2019.aspx.

CDC. (2019, October 25). *Polio Elimination in the United States.* Retrieved from Centers for Disease Control and Prevention: https://www.cdc.gov/polio/what-is-polio/polio-us.html.

CDC. (2016, May 3). *CDC: 1 in 3 Antibiotic Prescriptions Unnecessary.* Retrieved from Centers for Disease Control and Prevention: https://www.cdc.gov/media/releases/2016/ p0503-unnecessary-prescriptions.html.

Chase, L. (2019, July 25). *Generic Lyrica Now Approved for Nerve Pain.* Retrieved from GoodRx: https://www.goodrx.com/blog/ fda-approves-generic-lyrica/.

Ching, A. T. (2010). "A Dynamic Oligopoly Structural Model for the Prescription Drug Market after Patient Expiration." *International Economic Review, 51*(4), 1175–1207.

Ciociola, A., Cohen, L., and Kulkarni, P. (2014, May). "How Drugs Are Developed and Approved by the FDA: Current Process and Future Directions." *American Journal of Gastroenterology, 109*(5), 620–623. doi:10.1038/ajg.2013.407.

Crow, D. (2018, September 11). "Pharma Chief Defends 400% Drug Price as a 'Moral Requirement.'" Retrieved from *Financial Times:* https:// www.ft.com/content/48b0ce2c-b544-11e8-bbc3-ccd7de085ffe.

Dave, D. (2010, June). *Direct-to-Consumer Advertising in Pharmaceutical Markets: Effects on Demand and Prices.* Retrieved from Vox EU: https://voxeu.org/article/consumer-advert s-pharmaceuticals-impact-prices-and-sales.

Dearment, A. (2020, February 28). *Sorry, Martin Shkreli: FDA Approves First Generic Version of Daraprim.* Retrieved from MedCity: https://medcitynews.com/2020/02/sorry-marti n-shkreli-fda-approves-first-generic-version-of-daraprim/?rf=1.

Dearment, A. (b) (2020, January 28). *Martin Shkreli, His Former Company Thwarted Generic Competition against Toxoplasmosis Drug, FTC Says.* Retrieved from MedCity: https://medcitynews. com/2020/01/martin-shkreli-former-company-thwarted-ge neric-competition-against-toxoplasmosis-drug-ftc-says/?rf=1.

Dearment, A. (2018, August 9). "Report Blames Gaming of Patent System for High Drug Prices." *MedCity News*, p. 16.

DiMasi, J. A., Grabowski, H. G., and Hansen, R. W. (2016, May). "Innovation in the Pharmaceutical Industry: New Estimates of R&D Costs." *Journal of Health Economics, 47,* 20–33. doi:10.1016/j.jhealeco.2016.01.012.

Drettwan, J. J., and Kjos, A. L. (2019, June). "An Ethical Analysis of Pharmacy Benefit Manager (PBM) Practices." *Pharmacy, 7(2),* 65. doi:10.3390/pharmacy702006.

Duignan, B. (2013, September 16). *March of Dimes Foundation.* Retrieved from Britannica: https://www.britannica.com/topic/ March-of-Dimes-Foundation.

Dwyer, K. (2015, November 2). *The PBM Evolution.* Retrieved from Risk & Insurance: https://riskandinsurance.com/ the-pbm-evolution/.

Egan, M. (2016, August 29). How EpiPen Came to Symbolize Corporate Greed. Retrieved from CNN: https://money.cnn.

com/2016/08/29/investing/epipen-price-rise-history/index. html.

Egan, M. (b) (2016, August 25). EpiPen CEO: Blame the "Broken" System, Not Me. Retrieved from CNN: https://money.cnn. com/2016/08/25/investing/epipen-cost-ceo-lowers-price-mylan/index.html?iid=EL.

Ellyson, A. M., and Basu, A. (2018, March). *The New Prescription Drug Paradox: Pipeline Pressure and Rising Prices.* Retrieved from National Bureau of Economic Research: Working Paper 24387: https://www.nber.org/papers/w24387.

Emanuel, E. J. (2019, March 23). "Big Pharma's Go-To Defense of Soaring Drug Prices Doesn't Add Up." Retrieved from *The Atlantic:* https://www.theatlantic.com/health/archive/2019/03/dru g-prices-high-cost-research-and-development/585253/.

Engelberg, A. B. (2015, October 29). "How Government Policy Promotes High Drug Prices." Retrieved from *Health Affairs:* https:// www.healthaffairs.org/do/10.1377/hblog20151029.051488/full/.

Entis, L. (2019, April 9). "Why Does Medicine Cost So Much? Here's How Drug Prices Are Set." Retrieved from *Time:* https://time. com/5564547/drug-prices-medicine/.

FDA. (2020, October 2). *FDA List of Authorized Generic Drugs.* Retrieved from US Food & Drug Administration: https:// www.fda.gov/drugs/abbreviated-new-drug-application-anda/ fda-list-authorized-generic-drugs#:~:text=The%20term%20 %E2%80%9Cauthorized%20generic%E2%80%9D%20 drug,product%20as%20the%20branded%20product.

FDA. (b) (2020, February 28). *FDA Approves First Generic of Daraprim.* Retrieved from US Food & Drug Administration:

https://www.fda.gov/news-events/press-announcements/
fda-approves-first-generic-daraprim.

FDA. (c) (2020, February 5). *Frequently Asked Questions on Patents and Exclusivity.* Retrieved from US Food & Drug Administration: https://www.fda.gov/drugs/development-approval-process-drugs/frequently-asked-questions-patents-and-exclusivity#:~:text=Patents%20and%20exclusivity%20apply%20to,the%20statutory%20requirements%20are%20met.

FDA. (2012, September 10). *Kefauver-Harris Amendments Revolutionized Drug Development.* Retrieved from US Food & Drug Administration: https://www.fda.gov/consumers/consumer-updates/kefauver-harris-amendments-revolutionized-drug-development#:~:text=Once%20signed%20into%20law%20by,serious%20shortcomings%20at%20that%20time.

FDA. (n.d.). *Milestones in US Food and Drug Law History.* Retrieved from US Food & Drug Administration: https://www.fda.gov/about-fda/fdas-evolving-regulatory-powers/milestones-us-food-and-drug-law-history

Fiscella, K., Venci, J., Sanders, M., Lanigan, A. M., and Fortunua, R. J. (2019, May–June). "A Practical Approach to Reducing Patients' Prescription Costs." *Family Practice Management, 26*(3), 5–9. Retrieved from https://www.aafp.org/fpm/2019/0500/p5.html.

Frakt, A. (2018, November 12). "Something Happened to US Drug Costs in the 1990s." Retrieved from *New York Times:* https://www.nytimes.com/2018/11/12/upshot/why-prescription-drug-spending-higher-in-the-us.html.

Frakt, A. (2017, January 23). "Blame Technology, Not Longer Life Spans, for Health Spending Increases." Retrieved from *New*

York Times: https://www.nytimes.com/2017/01/23/upshot/ blame-technology-not-longer-life-spans-for-health-spending- increases.html.

Frank, R. G., Hicks, A., and Berndt, E. R. (2019, July). *The Price to Consumers of Generic Pharmaceuticals: Beyond the Headlines.* Retrieved from National Bureau of Economic Research: Working Paper 26120: https://www.nber.org/papers/w26120.

Freed, M., Neuman, T., and Cubanski, J. (2020, October 8). *10 FAQs on Prescription Drug Importation.* Retrieved from KFF: https://www.kff.org/medicare/issue-brief/10-faqs-on-pres cription-drug-importation/.

FTC. (2020). *The Antitrust Laws.* Retrieved from Federal Trade Commission: https://www.ftc.gov/tips-advice/ competition-guidance/guide-antitrust-laws/antitrust-laws.

FTC. (2010, January). *Pay-for-Delay: How Drug Company Pay- Offs Cost Consumers Billions.* Retrieved from Federal Trade Commission: https://www.ftc.gov/sites/default/files/ documents/reports/pay-delay-how-drug-company-pay- offs-cost-consumers-billions-federal-trade-commission-staff- study/100112payfordelayrpt.pdf.

Gill, L. L. (2020, January). "The Shocking Rise of Rx Drug Prices." *Consumer Reports,* pp. 38–48.

Greene, J. A., and Podolsky, S. H. (2012, October 18). "Reform, Regulation, and Pharmaceuticals: The Kefauver-Harris Amendments at 50." *New England Journal of Medicine, 367*(16), 1481–1483. doi:10.1056/NEJMp1210007.

Gregory, L. A. (2016, December 1). "Cashing Out: How Big Pharma Continues to Capitalize on the Antitrust Loophole Created in

FTC v. Actavis." *North Carolina Journal of Law & Technology,* *18*(5).

Hamblin, J. (2015, September 23). "Pharma Bro Is the Face of US Health Care." Retrieved from *The Atlantic:* https://www.theatlantic. com/health/archive/2015/09/martin-shkreli-in-the-mirror/406888/#:~:text=Pharma%20Bro%20Is%20the%20 Face%20of%20US%20Health%20Care&text=Discover%20 new%20ideas.,Rethink%20old%20assumptions.&text=In%20 what%20appears%20to%20be,more%20.

Harvard Health Publishing. (2020, April 10). *Which Drug for Erectile Dysfunction?* Retrieved from Harvard Health Publishing—Harvard Medical School: https://www.health.harvard.edu/ mens-health/which-drug-for-erectile-dysfunction.

Healthline. (2020, April). *The Long, Strange History of the EpiPen.* Retrieved from HealthLine: https://www.healthline.com/ health-news/strange-history-of-epipen.

Hemphill, T. A. (2016, July 6). *Eliminating Pharmaceutical Gray Markets.* Retrieved from RealClear Policy: https://www.realclearpolicy.com/ blog/2015/07/07/eliminating_pharmaceutical_gray_markets_ 1356.html#:~:text=Gray%20markets%20involve%20the%20 trading,because%20shortages%20facilitate%20price%2Dgouging.

Henka, D. (2018, April). Cutting Costs and Changing Habits with Reference Pricing. *Benefits Magazine,* pp. 46–51.

HHS. (2020, July 24). *Trump Administration Announces Historic Action to Lower Drug Prices for Americans.* Retrieved from HHS. gov: https://www.hhs.gov/about/news/2020/07/24/trum p-administration-announces-historic-action-lower-drug-prices-americans.html.

HHS. (2018, May). *American Patients First: The Trump Administration Blueprint to Lower Drug Prices and Reduce Out of Pocket Costs.* Retrieved from the US Department of Health & Human Services: https://www.hhs.gov/sites/default/files/AmericanPatientsFirst.pdf.

House Committee on Ways and Means. (2019, September). *A Painful Pill to Swallow: US vs. International Prescription Drug Prices.* Retrieved from Ways and Means Committee: https://waysandmeans.house.gov/sites/democrats.waysandmeans.house.gov/files/documents/US%20vs.%20International%20Prescription%20Drug%20Prices_0.pdf.

Howard, J. (2016, August 25). *EpiPen Cost Soars, but its' Not the Only Drug To.* Retrieved from CNN: https://www.cnn.com/2016/08/23/health/epipen-price-mylan-prescription-drugs-increase/index.html?iid=EL.

I-MAK. (2018, August). *Overpatented, Overpriced: How Excessive.* Retrieved from Medicines, Access, and Knowledge: http://www.i-mak.org/wp-content/uploads/2018/08/I-MAK-Overpatented-Overpriced-Report.pdf.

Ingram, R. A. (2015, July 19). "A Not-So-Transparent Attempt to Cap Drug Prices." Retrieved from *Wall Street Journal:* https://www.wsj.com/articles/a-not-so-transparent-attempt-to-cap-drug-prices-1437342475.

Jones, A. W. (2011, June). "Early Drug Discovery and the Rise of Pharmaceutical Industry." *Drug Testing and Analysis, 3*(6), 337–344. doi:10.1002/dta.301.

Jurney, C. (2016, July 28). "Global 2000: The World's Largest Drug and Biotech Companies." Retrieved from *Forbes:* https://www.

forbes.com/sites/corinnejurney/2016/05/27/2016-global-2000
-the-worlds-largest-drug-andbiotech-.

KFF. (2019, May 1). *Medicaid's Prescription Drug Benefit: Key Facts.*
Retrieved from KFF: https://www.kff.org/medicaid/fact-sheet/
medicaids-prescription-drug-benefit-key-facts/.

Kantarjian, H., Steensma, D., Sanjuan, J. R., Elshaug, A., and Light, D.
(2014). "High Cancer Drug Prices in the United States: Reasons and
Proposed Solutions." *Journal of Oncology Practice, 10*(4), e208–e211.

Khullar, D., and Bach, P. B. (2020, February 21). "*3 Actions Congress
Can Take to Reduce Drug Prices.*" Retrieved from *Harvard
Business Review:* https://hbr.org/2020/02/3-actions-congres
s-can-take-to-reduce-drug-prices.

Kirzinger, A., Neuman, T., Cubanski, J., and Brodie, M. (2019, August
9). *Data Note: Prescription Drugs and Older Adults.* Retrieved
from KFF: https://www.kff.org/health-reform/issue-brief/dat
a-note-prescription-drugs-and-older-adults/.

Klein, C. (2014, March 25). *8 Things You May Not Know about
Jonas Salk and the Polio Vaccine.* Retrieved from History.com:
https://www.history.com/news/8-things-you-may-not-kno
w-about-jonas-salk-and-the-polio-vaccine#:~:text=On%20
April%2012%2C%201955%2C%20the,asked%20who%20
owned%20the%20patent.

Kocot, S., McCutcheon, T., and White, R. (2019, January 22).
"Protected Class Policy Can Promote Both Patient Access and
Competition." Retrieved from *Health Affairs:* https://www.
healthaffairs.org/do/10.1377/hblog20190118.805215/full/.

Konrad, W. (2019, January 21). *Rx Drug Prices Continue to Rise:
Here's What You Can Do.* Retrieved from CBS News: https://

www.cbsnews.com/news/rx-drug-prices-continue-to-ris
e-heres-what-you-can-do/.

Kozarich, D. (2016, September 27). "Mylan's EpiPen Pricing Crossed Ethical Boundaries." Retrieved from *Fortune:* https://fortune. com/2016/09/27/mylan-epipen-heather-bresch/.

Long, C., and Hays, T. (2018, March 9). "'Pharma Bro' Gets 7 Years in Prison in Securities Fraud Case." Retrieved from AP News: https:// apnews.com/article/1edcd73fc8324e3b9285821a4c17c91e.

Longo, N. (2020, July 30). *Executive Order Threatens R&D When We Need It Most to Fight COVID-19.* Retrieved from Pharmaceutical Researcher and Manufacturers of America: https://catalyst.phrma.org/executiv e-order-threatens-rd-when-we-need-it-most-to-fight-covid-19?utm_ campaign=2020-q3-fed-fed_uns&utm_medium=pai-cpc-blg-ggl-adf&utm_source=ggl&utm_content=adv-adi-inf-tpv_scl-geo_be h-usa-all-nap-tgt-pai-cpc-blg-ggl-adf-EOSea.

Luthra, S. (2018, May 4). *"Pharma Bro" Shkreli Is in Prison, but Daraprim's Price Is Still High.* Retrieved from KHN: https:// khn.org/news/for-shame-pharma-bro-shkreli-is-in-prison-but -daraprims-price-is-still-high/.

Lyles, A. (2017, February). "Pharmacy Benefit Management Companies: Do They Create Value in the US Health Care System?" *PharmacoEconomics, 35*(5), 493–500. doi:10.1007/ s40273-017-0489-1.

Majerol, M., Tobert, J., and Damico, A. (2016, February 4). *Health Care Spending among Low-Income Households with and without Medicaid.* Retrieved from KFF: https://www.kff.org/medicaid/ issue-brief/health-care-spending-among-low-income-h ouseholds-with-and-without-medicaid/.

Marciarille, A. M. (2017, April). "The Prescription Drug Pricing Moment: Using Public Health Analysis to Clarify the Fair Competition Debate on Prescription Drug Pricing and Consumer Welfare." *The Journal of Law, Medicine & Ethics, 45*(1), 45–49. doi:10.1177/1073110517703323.

Mathew, R., Kilpatrick, L., and Garber, A. (2019, March). *The Real Price of Medications: A Survey of Variations in Prescription Drug Prices.* Retrieved from US PIRG Education Fund: https://uspirg.org/sites/pirg/files/reports/WEB_USP_Real-Price-Medications_030519.pdf.

McCarthy, R. (2017, Spring). *Early Pharmacy in America.* Retrieved from American Institute of the History of Pharmacy: https://aihp.org/wp-content/uploads/2018/08/1-Early-Pharmacy-in-America.pdf.

McKinnell, H. (2005). *A Call to Action: Taking Back Health Care for Future Generations.* New York, New York: McGraw Hill.

Medina, L., Sabo, S., and Vespa, J. (2020, February). *Living Longer: Historical and Projected Life Expectancy in the United States, 1960 to 2060.* Retrieved from US Census Bureau: https://www.census.gov/content/dam/Census/library/publications/2020/demo/p25-1145.pdf.

Meluch, A., and Oglesby, W. (2015). "Physician-Patient Communication Regarding Patients' Healthcare Costs in the US: A Systematic Review of the Literature." *Journal of Health Communication, 8*(2), 151–160.

Miyashiro, A. K. (2017, September 14). *Mylan's EpiPen Pricing Scandal.* Retrieved from Seven Pillars Institute: https://sevenpillarsinstitute.org/mylans-epipen-pricing-scandal/.

Molinder, H. (1994, October). "The Development of Cimetidine: 1964–1976. A Human Story." *Clinical Gastroenterology and Hepatology, 19*(3), 248–254.

Morse, S. (2019, March 20). *High Price of Drugs Is Biggest Issue in Prescription Adherence, Physicians Say.* Retrieved from Healthcare Finance: https://www.healthcarefinancenews.com/news/high-price-drugs-biggest-issue-prescription-adherence-physicians-say.

Mui, K. (2019, September 16). *Generic Doxycycline Still Too Expensive? Here Are Some Alternatives.* Retrieved from GoodRx: https://www.goodrx.com/blog/alternatives-to-doxycycline-a-common-drug-with-a-complicated-past/.

Nagle, T. T., Hogan, J., and Zale, J. (2017). *The Strategy and Tactics of Pricing.* London, United Kingdom: Routledge.

OCED. (2019). *Pharmaceutical Spending.* Retrieved from OCED Data: https://data.oecd.org/healthres/pharmaceutical-spending.htm.

Ohn, J. A., and Kaltenboeck, A. (2019, August). *Evolving Medicaid Coverage Policy and Rebates.* Retrieved from AMA Journal of Ethics: https://journalofethics.ama-assn.org/article/evolving-medicaid-coverage-policy-and-rebates/2019-08.

Oliver, T. R., Lee, P. R., and Lipton, H. L. (2004, June). "A Political History of Medicare and Prescription Drug Coverage." *The Milbank Quarterly, 82*(2), 283–354. doi:10.1111/j.0887-378X.2004.00311.x.

Ornstein, C., Weber, T., and Grochowski, R. (2019, October 17). *We Found over 700 Doctors Who Were Paid More than a Million Dollars by Drug and Medical Device Companies.* Retrieved from

ProPublica: https://www.propublica.org/article/we-found-over-700-doctors-who-were-paid-more-than-a-million-dollars-by-drug-and-medical-device-companies.

Orwig, S. (2018, September 7). *The 340B Drug Pricing Controversy, Explained.* Retrieved from the Advisory Board: https://www.advisory.com/daily-briefing/2017/12/12/340b-explained.

Osborn, R., Squires, D., Doty, M. M., Sarnak, DO, and Schneider, E. C. (2016, November 16). *In a New Survey of 11 Countries, US Adults Still Struggle with Access to and Affordability of Health Care.* Retrieved from The Commonwealth Fund: https://www.commonwealthfund.org/publications/journal-article/2016/nov/new-survey-11-countries-us-adults-still-struggle-access-and.

Owles, E. (2017, June 22). "The Making of Martin Shkreli as 'Pharma Bro.'" Retrieved from *New York Times:* https://www.nytimes.com/2017/06/22/business/dealbook/martin-shkreli-pharma-bro-drug-prices.html.

Palmer, B. (2014, April 13). *Jonas Salk: Good at Virology, Bad at Economics.* Retrieved from Slate: https://slate.com/technology/2014/04/the-real-reasons-jonas-salk-didnt-patent-the-polio-vaccine.html.

Panteli, Dimitra, et al. (2016). *Pharmaceutical Regulation in 15 European Countries.* (D. Panteli, and R. Busse, Eds.) Retrieved from Health Systems in Transition—European Observatory on Health Systems and Policies: https://www.euro.who.int/__data/assets/pdf_file/0019/322444/HiT-pharmaceutical-regulation-15-European-countries.pdf?ua=1.

Pearl, R. (2019, June 14). *The Ethics behind the World's Most Expensive Medication.* Retrieved from KevinMD: https://www.

kevinmd.com/blog/2019/06/the-ethics-behind-the-world
s-most-expensive-medication.html.

Pearl, R. (2018, September 24). "The Immorality of Prescription Drug
Pricing in America." Retrieved from *Forbes:* https://www.forbes.
com/sites/robertpearl/2018/09/24/nostrum/#132f9b474fb1.

Penn Wharton. (2016, June 27). *Mortality in the United States:
Past, Present, and Future.* Retrieved from Budget Model—
University of Pennsylvania: https://budgetmodel.wharton.
upenn.edu/issues/2016/1/25/mortality-in-the-united-state
s-past-present-and-future.

PharmaPhorum. (2020, September 1). *A History of the Pharmaceutical
Industry.* Retrieved from PharmaPhorum: https://
pharmaphorum.com/r-d/a_history_of_the_pharmaceutical_
industry/.

Pratt, C. (2017, January 16). *3 Blockbuster Drugs That Changed
the Market.* Retrieved from Biotech Investing News:
https://investingnews.com/daily/life-science-investing/
pharmaceutical-investing/3-blockbuster-drugs-changed-the-
market/#:~:text=Tagamet%20was%20the%20world's%20
first,treats%20ulcers%20and%20gastrointestinal%20problems.

Prihoda, C. (2017). *A Case for Care and the Costs of Capitalism: The
Ethics of Prescription Drug Pricing.* Retrieved from Philosophy
Honors Papers: https://digitalcommons.conncoll.edu/
philhp/11.

Roche, D. (2020, September 29). "Big Pharma Backs Joe Biden,
but People Don't Think He'll Fix Drug Pricing." Retrieved from
Newsweek: https://www.newsweek.com/big-pharma-joe-bide
n-fix-drug-pricing-1534809.

Rosenbaum, L., and Shrank, W. H. (2013, August 22). "Taking Our Medicine: Improving Adherence in the Accountability Era." *New England Journal of Medicine, 369*(8), 694–695. doi:10.1056/NEJMp1307084.

Saganowsky, E. (2019, July 29). *Mylan CEO Bresch Set to Exit after Years of Controversy—And One Last Big Deal.* Retrieved from Fierce Pharma: https://www.fiercepharma.com/pharma/following-eventful-8-years-mylan-ceo-heather-bresch-set-to-retire-after-upjohn-deal.

Sagonowksy, E. (2018, November 28). *Pfizer Wins Blockbuster Lyrica Patent Extension to Safeguard Sales till June.* Retrieved from Fierce Pharma: https://www.fiercepharma.com/pharma/pfizer-wins-blockbuster-patent-extension-for-lyrica-exclusivity-now-stretches-until-june.

Salk, J. (1955, April 12). Interview with Edward R. Murrow (E. R. Murrow, interviewer).

Sarnak, D. O., Squires, D., and Bishop, S. (2017, October 5). *Paying for Prescription Drugs around the World: Why Is the US an Outlier?* Retrieved from The Commonwealth Fund: https://www.commonwealthfund.org/publications/issue-briefs/2017/oct/paying-prescription-drugs-around-world-why-us-outlier.

Sarpatwari, A., DeBello, J., Zakarian, M., Najafzadeh, M., and Kesselheim, A. S. (2019). "Competition and Price among Brand-Name Drugs in the Same Class: A Systematic Review of the Evidence." *PLoS Medicine, 16*(7), e1002872. doi:10.1371/journal.pmed.1002872.

Schondelmeyer, S. W., and Purvis, L. (2019, November). *Brand Name Drug Prices Increase More than Twice as Fast as Inflation*

in 2018. Retrieved from AARP: https://www.aarp.org/
content/dam/aarp/ppi/2019/11/brand-name-drug-price
s-increase-more-than-twice-as-fast-as-inflation.doi.10.26419-
2Fppi.00073.005.pdf.

Schultz, L., Lowe, T. J., Srinavasan, A., and Pugliese, G. (2014, October). "Economic Impact of Redundant Antimicrobial Therapy in US Hospitals." *Infection Control and Hospital Epidemiology, 35*(10), 1229–1235. doi:10.1086/678066.

Seeley, E., and Kesselheim, A. S. (2019, March 26). *Pharmacy Benefit Managers: Practices, Controversies and What Lies Ahead.* Retrieved from The Commonwealth Fund: https://www. commonwealthfund.org/publications/issue-briefs/2019/ mar/pharmacy-benefit-managers-practices-controversie s-what-lies-ahead.

Smith, J. S. (1991). *Patenting the Sun: Polio and the Salk Vaccine.* New York, NY: Morrow.

Sorter, A. W. (2013, December 2). *Researchers and Advocates Work Together to Advance Glioblastoma Understanding and Treatment.* Retrieved from Cure Today: https://www.curetoday.com/view/ researchers-and-advocates-work-together-to-advance-gliobla stoma-understanding-and-treatment.

Squires, D., and Anderson, C. (2015, October 8). *US Health Care from a Global Perspective: Spending, Use of Services, Prices and Health in 13 Countries.* Retrieved from The Commonwealth Fund: http:// www.commonwealthfund.org/publications/issue-briefs/2015/ oct/ushealth-.

Sullivan, T. (2020, September 20). *President Trump Signs "Most Favored Nation Price" Executive Order on Drug Pricing.*

Retrieved from Policy & Medicine: https://www.policymed. com/2020/09/president-trump-signs-most-favored-nation-pri ce-executive-order-on-drug-pricing.html.

Swanson, A. (2015, June 30). "How New Drugs Helping Millions of Americans Live Longer Are Also Making Them Go Broke." Retrieved from *Washington Post:* https://www. washingtonpost.com/news/wonk/wp/2015/06/30/how-ne w-drugs-helping-millions-of-americans-live-longer-are-a lso-making-them-go-broke/.

Tantibanchachai, C. (2014, April 1). *US Regulatory Response to Thalidomide (1950–2000).* Retrieved from The Embryo Project Encyclopedia: https://embryo.asu.edu/pages/us-regulator y-response-thalidomide-1950-2000

Tobbell, D. (2012). *Pills, Power and Policy: The Struggle for Drug Reform in Cold War America and Its Consequences.* Los Angeles, CA: University of California Press.

Totenberg, N. (2020, November 10). "Will Supreme Court Invalidate Obamacare a Decade after It Was Enacted?" Retrieved from NPR's *Morning Edition:* https://www.npr. org/2020/11/10/932441334/will-supreme-court-invalidate-o bamacare-a-decade-after-it-was-enacted.

Trump, D. J. (2020, September 13). *Executive Order on Lowering Drug Prices by Putting America First.* Retrieved from WhiteHouse. gov: https://www.whitehouse.gov/presidential-actions/executiv e-order-lowering-drug-prices-putting-america-first-2/.

Ubl, S. J. (2020, September 13). *PhRMA Statement on Most Favored Nation Executive Order.* Retrieved from Pharmaceutical Research and Manufacturers of America: https://phrma.

org/Press-Release/PhRMA-Statement-on-Most-Favore
d-Nation-Executive-Order.

van der Gronde, T., Uyl-de Groot, C., and Pieters, T. (2017, August). "Addressing the Challenge of High-Priced Prescription Drugs in the Era of Precision Medicine: A Systematic Review of Drug Life Cycles, Therapeutic Drug Markets and Regulatory Frameworks." *PLoS ONE, 12*(8), 1–34. doi:10.1371/journal.pone.0182613.

Vallenas, N. (2020, May 23). *The Dilemma of Pharmaceutical Promotion Practices: A Conversation with Dr. Aaron Kesselheim.* Retrieved from Harvard Health Policy Review: http://www.hhpronline. org/articles/2020/5/23/the-dilemma-of-pharmaceutical-promotion-practices-a-conversation-with-dr-aaron-kesselheim.

Van Zee, A. (2009, February). "The Promotion and Marketing of OxyContin: Commercial Triumph, Public Health Tragedy." *American Journal of Public Health, 99*(2), 221–227. doi:10.2105/AJPH.2007.131714.

Waldrop, T., and Rapfogel, N. (2020, October 15). *Too Little, Too Late: Trump's Prescription Drug Executive Order Does Not Help Patients.* Retrieved from Center for American Progress: https://www.americanprogress.org/issues/healthcare/news/2020/10/15/491425/little-late-trumps-prescriptio n-drug-executive-order-not-help-patients/.

Weatherall, M. (1990). *In Search of a Cure: A History of Pharmaceutical Discovery.* Oxford: Oxford University Press.

Weber, T., and Ornstein, C. (2013, March 11). *Dollars for Docs Mints a Millionaire.* Retrieved from ProPublica: https://www.propublica.org/article/dollars-for-docs-mints-a-millionaire.

World Health Organization. (2009, August). *Direct-to-Consumer Advertising under Fire.* Retrieved from World Health Organization: https://www.who.int/bulletin/volumes/87/8/09-040809/en/#:~:text=Direct%2Dto%2Dconsumer%20advertising%20of,(long%20format%20television%20commercials).

Wouters, O. J., Kanavos, P. G., and McKee, M. (2017). Comparing Generic Drug Markets in Europe and the United States: Prices, Volumes, and Spending. *The Milbank Quarterly, 95*(3), 554–601.

Yu, N. L., Helms, Z., and Bach, P. S. (2017, March 7). "R&D Costs for Pharmaceutical Companies Do Not Explain Elevated Drug Prices." Retrieved from *Health Affairs:* https://www.healthaffairs.org/do/10.1377/hblog20170307.059036/full/.

INDEX

drug lag, 52
Drug Price Competition and Patent
  Term Restoration Act (1984), 52,
  79, 93
drug production, shifts in, 11
drug supply chain
  determining actual value of drug and
    determining "fair" pricing as
    differing along, 136
  disruptions in, 84
  as having many stakeholders, 136
  interference along, 67
  little public information as available
    concerning financial transac-
    tions between participants in, 60
  as not driven by competitive market
    forces, 75
  recommendation for public disclo-
    sure at each step of, 173
  recommendation for requiring
    greater price transparency
    along, 183
drugs. *See also* cancer medications; generic drugs; *specific drugs*
  blockbuster drugs, 16, 18, 111, 149,
    151, 152, 185
  importation of, 165–166, 177
  "me-too drugs," 13
  multiple sclerosis drugs, 158
  "novel" pharmaceuticals, 21,
    122–123
  "orphan drugs," 70, 141
  as prolonging life, 48
  "protected" class of drugs under
    Medicare Part D, 59–60
  specialty drugs, 18, 37, 48, 57–58, 67,
    99, 110, 111, 171
  synthetic drugs, 5
  three-stage period/journey of, 174
duloxetine (Cymbalta), 191

E

Eli Lilly
  as bringing lawsuit against "show-
    me-the-price" rule, 169
  collaborative production of insulin
    by, 9
  development of Prozac, 16
  founding of, 6
  as generic drug manufacturer, 14–15
  as one of "old-line" pharmaceutical
    companies, 10
Ellyson, A. M., 67
Emanuel, Ezekiel, 55, 168–169
England, as exporter of most medicines
  early on, 7
EpiPen, outrage over, 125–132
EpiPen4Schools program, 126,
  129, 131
Epsom salts, 5, 6
erectile dysfunction drugs, 55, 145,
  156, 180
ERP (external reference pricing) system, 154, 155, 159
ethical conflicts, of making money
  from selling health care products, 12
ethical models
  choices model, 139, 140
  common good model, 139, 140
  exceptions model, 139, 140
  justice model, 139, 140
  utility model (utilitarianism),
    139, 140
  virtue model, 139, 140
  "ethical pricing," 130, 135, 136–137
ethics
  and morality of pharmaceuticals and
    prices, 120–147
  versus profit, 138–147

evergreening, 64, 86–89, 176, 182

exclusion lists, 33–34, 140

executive orders, use of by President Trump in attempt to lower drug prices, 164–166, 167, 177

Express Scripts, as one of three dominant PBMs, 34

external reference pricing (ERP) system, 154, 155, 159

F

FDA (Food and Drug Administration). See Food and Drug Administration (FDA)

Federal Trade Commission Act (1914), 68

Federal Trade Commission (FTC)
actions of that would address problem of high prescription prices, 176
charges against Vyera Pharmaceuticals, xiii
as condemning reverse-payment schemes, 93
on monopolization, 68–69
as needing to crack down on shady practices by pharmaceutical manufacturers, 182
as needing to step in to more aggressively enforce antitrust laws, 89
number of generic entries as impacting overall price competition according to, 94
theory of toward competition and antimonopolistic practices as having flaws, 94

fibromyalgia syndrome (FMS), treatment for, 86–88

fine chemical manufacturers, 10

Finland, pricing of drugs in, 155

Fiscella, K., 187

Fleming, Alexander, 9

Food, Drug and Cosmetic Act (1938), 10, 49, 51

Food and Drug Administration (FDA)
actions of that would address problem of high prescription prices, 176
approval of EpiPen by, 125, 126, 127
approval of first generic version of Daraprim (pyrimethamne), xiii
approval of Zolgensma by, 141, 142
"impurities" rule, 133, 134
odds of having drug approved for sale by, 25
Pure Food and Drugs Act (1906), 8
role of regarding drugs, 13, 14, 17, 18, 27, 30, 50, 51–52, 54, 55, 70, 72, 81, 82, 84, 86, 88, 89, 91, 92, 93, 174, 175, 180, 182, 184
as strengthening DTC advertising from drug companies, 2, 29

formularies, 32, 37, 59, 64, 113–114, 150

Frank, R. G., 95

"free market" concept/approach, 13, 22, 25, 40, 63–65, 66–67, 68, 81, 149, 180

Friedrich Bayer Company, 5

FTC (Federal Trade Commission). See Federal Trade Commission (FTC)

FTC v. Actavis, 93

G

gag clauses/orders, 34, 140, 155, 163–164, 169

GBM (glioblastoma multiforme), 144–145

collaborative production of penicillin by, 9
development of Lyrica by, 86–88
founding of, 6
as one of largest fine chemical manufacturer, 10
"Pharma Bro," as Shkreli nickname, xi
pharmaceutical companies
as contributors to higher drug prices,
24–31
difficulty for smaller companies to
compete against Big Pharma,
53–54
in-house laboratories of, 8
justification for high prices by, 25
marketing costs of, 27–30
as not liking generic counterparts, 78
as operating in atmosphere of monopoly pricing, 30
profit margins of, 145
as promoting heavily and directly to
physicians and prescribers, 41
research costs of, 24–27
shaming of into lowering prices,
168–169
pharmaceutical industry
as challenging presidential executive
orders in court, 169, 177
contributions to Biden campaign, 172
contributions to Trump campaign, 172
as highly opaque regarding pricing
strategies, 72
as high-risk, high-cost industry, 25
little as "competitive" about, 75
as not fitting a capitalistic structure, 63
as operating within highly specialized
distribution environment, 37–38

percent of revenues for marketing
and creating awareness for specific drug brands, 190
Pharmaceutical Manufacturers
Association (PMA), 22, 80
Pharmaceutical Researcher and
Manufacturers of America
(PhRMA), 167, 179
pharmaceuticals
as compared to biologics, 18
early ones as mostly natural, 3–4
factors that determine a country's
spending on, 152
as following their own pricing
rules, 64
getting a drug from manufacturer to
market, 23
history of, 3–11
history of high costs of, 1–2
"novel" pharmaceuticals, 21
per capita spending on, 150–151
regulation of, 8, 10
US spending on, 17–18
pharmacies, separation of from medical
practices, 7
Pharmacist Code of Ethics, 140
pharmacology, establishment of, 5
pharmacy benefit managers (PBMs)
as contributors to higher drug prices,
31–35
potential changes by that could address problem of high prescription prices, 178–179
rebates to from drug manufacturers,
31–33, 34, 66, 136, 183
PhRMA (Pharmaceutical Researcher
and Manufacturers of America),
167, 179
Physician Code of Ethics, 140
physicians

as contributors to higher drug prices, 40–47

as incentivized by pharmaceutical manufacturers, 67

as rarely having any direct incentive to select most cost-effective treatments, 67

role of in finding solutions to high prescription prices, 185–189

pipeline pressure, impact of on drug costs, 67

plant alkaloids, identification of, 5

PMA (Pharmaceutical Manufacturers Association), 22, 80

poliomyelitis/polio, 121–124

Pravachol (pravastatin), 84

pregabalin (Lyrica), 86–88, 91

prescribers, role of in finding solutions to high prescription prices, 185–189

prescriptions, pharmaceuticals as beginning with, 64

price controls, 12, 22, 102, 105, 111, 149, 150, 153, 157–160, 163, 174

price fixing, 11, 12

price mandates, 168

price matching, 72

pricing. *See also* "list prices"

of brand-name drugs, xv

contributors to higher drug prices, 23–61

efforts to reform, 22–23

"ethical pricing," 130, 135, 136–137

"just pricing," x, 135, 136, 137, 145, 156

little standardization in, 38

no federal law or regulation keeping drug prices in check, 21

outcome-based pricing, 173

reference pricing, as idea for solution to high prescription prices, 107, 173, 187–188

transparency of. *See* transparency, of pricing

pricing strategy tests, 129–130, 132, 143

product hopping, 89, 176, 182

profit, ethics versus, 138–147

ProPublica, on doctors on Big Pharma payroll, 41–42

"protected" class of drugs under Medicare Part D, 59–60

purchasing power, consolidation and application of, 181

Purdue Pharma, manufacturer of OxyContin, 44–45

Pure Food and Drugs Act (1906), 8

pyrimethamine (Daraprim), xi, xii, xiii, 18, 24, 91, 94

Q

quinine, 3

R

rebates

to the government from pharmaceutical manufacturers, 112. *See also* Medicaid Drug Rebate Program (MDRP)

from pharmaceutical manufacturers to PBMs, 31–33, 34, 66, 136, 183

from private insurers to members, 179

redundant treatment, costs of, 44

reference pricing, as idea for solution to high prescription prices, 107, 173, 187–188

research
    as competitive strategy among pharmaceutical companies, 8
    costs of, 24–27
    during World War II, 10
retail pharmacies, as contributors to higher drug prices, 37–39
reverse payments, a.k.a. "pay-for-delay" agreements, 92–93, 156, 176, 182
Richardson-Merrell, distributor of thalidomide, 50, 51
Rite Aid, on generic pricing, 39
Roberts, Jonathan, 7
RxSaver (app), 187

S

Salk, Jonas, 121–122, 123, 124
Sarnak, D. O., 151–152
School Access to Emergency Epinephrine Act (2013), 126
Scully, James H., Jr., 42
Senate Subcommittee on Antitrust and Monopoly, Kefauver hearings, 12–14
senior citizens
    drug discontinuance and nonadherence by, 109–110
    and prescription drugs, 98–111
Sertuner, Fredrich, 4
Sharp & Dohme, Merck merger with, 11
Sherman Antitrust Act (1890), 68, 69, 92
Shkreli, Martin, xi–xii, xiii, 18, 24, 146
"show-me-the-price" rule, 169–170
Simpson, James Young, 5
simvastatin, 191
SingleCare (app), 187
"single-source" fallacy, as contributor to higher drug prices, 60

SMA (spinal muscular atrophy), Zolgensma as cure for, 141, 142, 144
Smith, Kline & French
    development of cimetidine (Tagamet), 16
    as one of "old-line" pharmaceutical companies, 10
    research on peptic ulcers, 15–16
society, impacts of high prescription prices on, 117–119
solutions (to high prescription prices)
    consumers' role in finding, 189–193
    enforcement of antitrust laws, 176
    government's role in finding, 179–185
    incentives, 173, 174–175
    need for holistic approach to, 173–174, 178
    outcome-based pricing, 173
    patent reform legislation, 173
    physicians'/prescribers' role in finding, 185–189
    reference pricing, 107, 173, 187–188
    transparency of pricing, 167, 168, 173, 183, 196
Sovaldi/Harvoni, 2, 16, 57, 136, 142
specialty drugs
    Biden's proposal to form new arm of HHS to assess value of new ones, 171
    biologics as classified as, 37
    as contributors to higher drug prices, 57–58, 67
    defined, 48
    as keeping older people alive for longer, 99, 110
    Medicaid as paying disproportionate share of certain ones, 111

ABOUT THE AUTHOR

Dr. Richard George Boudreau is a maxillofacial surgeon, bioethicist, attorney at law, and forensic expert who serves on the faculty of the U.C.L.A. Department of Oral & Maxillofacial Surgery. His extensive academic credentials include BS, MA, MBA, DDS, MD, JD, PhD, PsyD degrees and several fellowships. He has dutifully and tirelessly volunteered in several academic teaching capacities and committees over many years and has passionate interest in health care, ethics, law, theology, philosophy, education, public policy. He especially enjoys authoring articles and books, researching and teaching this scholarly and profound discipline. He is a prolific bioethics lecturer, author, columnist with regular media contributions, and a regular contributor to several newspapers and magazines. His books include: *Bioethics Perspective of the Feasibility and Implementation of an Existential Psychoanalytic Praxis Addressing End-of-Life Care in the Elderly; Incorporating Bioethics Education into School Curriculums; US Universal Health Care in 2020; Medical Error, Ethics, and Apology.* One of his alma maters, Pepperdine Univ., honored him in 2011 with the 'George Award' which is awarded to recipients who "exemplify integrity, stewardship, courage, and compassion, while enriching the ever changing world through superior skills and spirit."

www.ingramcontent.com/pod-product-compliance
Lightning Source LLC
Chambersburg PA
CBHW021356210526
45463CB00001B/116